Animal-Assisted Therapy with Dogs

Springer Nature More Media App

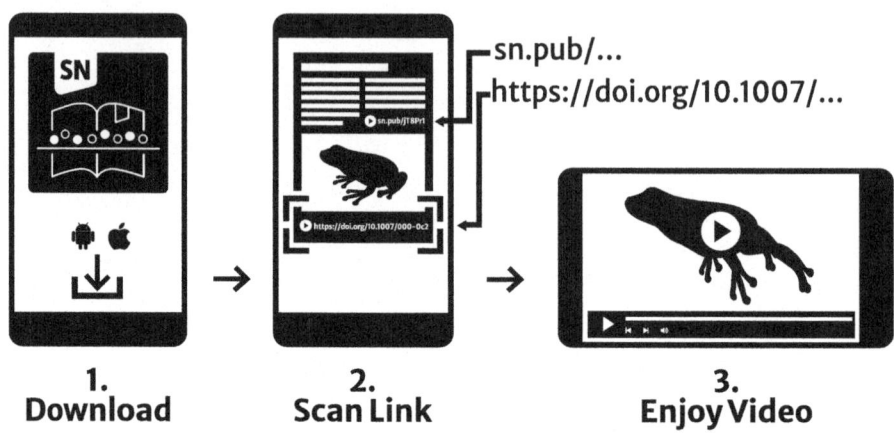

sn.pub/...
https://doi.org/10.1007/...

1.
Download

2.
Scan Link

3.
Enjoy Video

Support: customerservice@springernature.com

Katharina Blesch

Animal-Assisted Therapy with Dogs

Basics, Animal Ethics and Practice of Therapeutic Work

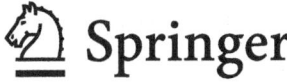 Springer

Katharina Blesch
Herrischried, Germany

This work contains media enhancements, which are displayed with a "play" icon. Material in the print book can be viewed on a mobile device by downloading the Springer Nature "More Media" app available in the major app stores. The media enhancements in the online version of the work can be accessed directly by authorized users.

ISBN 978-3-662-67964-7   ISBN 978-3-662-67965-4   (eBook)
https://doi.org/10.1007/978-3-662-67965-4

Translation from the German language edition: "Tiergestützte Therapie mit Hunden" by Katharina Blesch, © Springer-Verlag GmbH Deutschland, ein Teil von Springer Nature 2020. Published by Springer Berlin Heidelberg. All Rights Reserved.

This Springer imprint is published by the registered company Springer-Verlag GmbH, DE, part of Springer Nature.
The registered company address is: Heidelberger Platz 3, 14197 Berlin, Germany

In memory of Cleo, whose nature will always remain a model for me.

Preface

"Any glimpse into the life of an animal quickens our own
and makes it so much the larger and better in every way"
(Muir in Hatkoff, 2009, p. 176)

There is hardly a quote that would better describe why I live and work with animals. Every interaction with an animal leaves traces in my memory, and every deeper interaction changes me. As long as I can remember, animals have been an important part of my life, and with each phase of development, the presence of animals in my life has expanded and solidified.

In my childhood, budgerigar, guinea pig, and dog were my pets and friends. In my youth in Italy, I became involved with animal protection. A teacher at my school initiated contact for some of us students with a large animal shelter on the outskirts of Milan. This shelter housed about 400 dogs. From then on, I had a small black godchild dog, Pepe, and regularly took him and his kennel neighbor, the shepherd mix bitch Stella, for walks with my mother. The already more bad than right conditions of the dogs worsened over time. Dogs disappeared one by one, which in our naivety at the time only puzzled us, as it seemed unlikely to us that these dogs had been placed. If at all, puppies were placed from time to time, but even that was a rarity. So where were all these big dogs? The owner of the shelter at this time invented various explanations. A nice caretaker, who took care of Pepe and Stella and the other dogs, assured me that he would especially look after Pepe and Stella. However, things turned out differently, and when we came for a walk one morning, Stella was no longer there. Pepe was alone in his kennel, panting and barking in panic. The caretaker said that Stella had simply been gone in the morning when he came to feed—like all the other dogs that had disappeared so far. The owner of the shelter then indulged in changing excuses: Stella had been adopted. Oh no, Stella had had surgery on her snout and was still in the clinic. No, Stella had unfortunately died during the operation. Confronted with our accusations and tears, she finally threatened to set her Doberman on us if we did not leave the shelter immediately. So we took the frightened Pepe and left. We reported the incident to the Carabinieri, the responsible police. The caretaker and other people did the same, so that it finally led to charges and subsequently a court case against the owner of the shelter. It turned out that all the dogs that had disappeared over the last few months had been killed and buried in the adjacent forest. Over 300 dogs met this end. The reason for this was the money that the owner received for each dog and that she continued to collect after the unofficial disappearance of the dogs.

Pepe lived with us for another three years before we had to put him to sleep with heavy hearts at the age of about thirteen. He had spent nine years in this shelter and had been physically marked by it. His nature, however, had not been clouded by all this. Pepe was a cheerful dog, full of trust and affection towards our family. And Pepe was grateful. He integrated into everything without any problems, went on trips, stayed alone, never caused any difficulties, just wanted to be and to please, without being submissive. Without diminishing my other great dogs, Pepe is still for me the epitome of resilience and a loyal companion.

Stella's disappearance was the sad occasion for my involvement in animal welfare and animal ethics, which began in my adolescence. To this day, these are my main concerns. With the start of my training as a diploma psychologist, animal behavior therapist, animal trainer, and animal-assisted therapist, and my entry into professional life, these concerns expanded. There was an added desire to promote the understanding through working with animals in the context of animal-assisted therapy that the protection and enhancement of animal welfare does not have to contradict working with them, but on the contrary, that animal welfare and animal-assisted therapy can go hand in hand and can mutually reinforce each other.

My animal companions make this work possible. Currently, I live and work with the mixed-breed dogs Giulio, Cleo, and Toni, who come from animal welfare. Along with them, the rabbits Alice and Frederick and the guinea pigs Fritz and Philip, who also come from animal welfare, live with me and are also partially used by me in therapy. My horse Marie was also previously used by me in therapeutic work, but is now enjoying her well-deserved retirement.

I cannot and do not want to imagine my private and professional life without animals. The experiences with them have shaped me and are an incentive for further development and improvement today. In relation to this book, the animals are the protagonists—and hopefully the beneficiaries. Beneficiaries insofar as this book should help to overcome the separation between animal welfare and animal-assisted therapy. We do not have to choose between either *good for humans* or *good for the animal*—both are possible together if we leave the beaten path, open ourselves to new things, and approach the matter correctly. I describe what this can look like exactly on the following pages.

Katharina Blesch

Acknowledgment

My greatest and most important thanks go to my parents, Drs. Kyra and Rainer Blesch. Not only this book, but also most of my other activities with and around animals would not be possible without their constant support. My projects have always been unconditionally accepted and promoted by them. And all my animals have a second home with my parents and are always welcome—no matter what condition, no matter what difficult behaviors, whether fully trained or just fresh from the animal shelter.

I would also like to thank my partner Maurizio Barbagallo at this point for his participation in the videos and his support in everyday life.

I would like to thank my dear friend Eva-Irina Mühleck for her support and practical help in the final phase of the book.

And I thank the people who had a lasting influence on me during my training and my first steps in the animal-assisted area. These are Alessandra Cova, psychologist at the AGRES Hippotherapy Center in Rescaldina, and Claudio Villa, head of the ASOM rehabilitation project at the Bollate prison near Milan.

Furthermore, I am grateful to my former superiors, Dr. Martin Gerken and Dr. Christian Klesse, who made the implementation of my ideas possible through their openness and the creation of space.

Contents

Animal-Assisted Therapy— Basics and My Personal Understanding of this Discipline

1

Contents

Abstract

This chapter introduces animal-assisted therapy as a discipline—after presenting the past and the current state, the focus is primarily on the necessary further development of this discipline. As a basis, the exact definition of animal-assisted therapy is discussed first, and correct terms are introduced in this context. For further understanding of this field, an overview of the various effective factors and the history of animal-assisted therapy is provided. In the next step, using my own work method as an example, a further development of animal-assisted therapy is described, which takes new paths and addresses ethical questions.

K. Blesch, *Animal-Assisted Therapy with Dogs*, https://doi.org/10.1007/978-3-662-67965-4_1

1.1   Definition and Terminology

Animals[1] play a pivotal role in all areas of human life. They are pets to humans, serve as livestock and food, were formerly used as working animals and in more recent times are being trained and educated to assist humans in various areas. On television, they are popular figures and entertainers, in art and literature they are symbols, projection surfaces, possibilities for visualization. And this is not just a recent development.

Even in cave paintings, animals were not only present, but the central motif of humans. Art historian Seeberg assumes that even in cave paintings, the depiction of animals served as a mirror for humans: "we find something of ourselves in them" (Seeberg, 2008, p. 33). Later on we will discuss where this old and strong connection of humans to animals comes from. To summarize at this point: Animals are present wherever humans are—and have always been.

It is therefore not surprising that animals are also used in human therapy. This use of an animal in the therapy of a human is referred to as *Animal-Assisted Therapy*. There are now many different definitions and descriptions of this term. A common and concise definition of animal-assisted therapy is as follows:

▶ **Common Definition of Animal-Assisted Therapy** "Animal-assisted therapy refers to all measures in which the targeted use of an animal is intended to have positive effects on the experience and behavior of humans." (Gatterer quoted after Pottmann-Knapp, 2013, p. 40)

However, animal-assisted therapy is not yet a uniform form of therapy. This is partly due to the fact that the term animal therapist is not yet a protected professional title. Nevertheless, representatives of this discipline have formulated certain conditions that are not legally binding, but are generally accepted. These conditions are intended to standardize the discipline and strengthen its credibility. However, there are differences in the formulations of the various umbrella organizations. In the following, I formulate the definition of animal-assisted therapy freely according to the definition of ESAAT (=European Society for Animal-Assisted Therapy), as it includes all central aspects:

▶ **Conditions of Animal-Assisted Therapy (freely according to ESAAT, 2012)** Animal-assisted therapy …

---

[1] Since humans belong to the animal kingdom, the correct term here should be "non-human animals". For better readability, however, this term is not used here and in the following, and the term "animals" is used as a shorthand when referring to non-human animals.

- includes consciously planned educational, psychological, and social integrative offerings with animals, in which participants interact with animals, communicate about animals, and/or work for animals
- has as potential target groups *people of all ages with limitations or support needs in the areas of cognition, psyche, and/or motor skills*
- can also be used *preventively* for health promotion
- is always carried out by a *professional* in animal-assisted therapy, i.e., by someone who …
- has a therapeutic basic profession (doctor, psychologist, occupational therapist, etc.),
- has learned to integrate animals into the therapy he offers (for example, as part of a training recognized by ESAAT),
- and is well acquainted with the type of animal used
- has a concrete and patient-specific *therapy goal*
- is *documented* in terms of its progress

This definition, freely formulated according to ESAAT, is, in my understanding, the best and most concise description of animal-assisted therapy.

The conditions mentioned in the definition distinguish animal-assisted therapy from other areas of animal use. Such as *activities with animals*. To speak of animal-assisted therapy, the offerings, as described above, must be carried out by a professional in animal-assisted therapy, have concrete and participant-specific goals, and have to be documented in their progress. All activities in which animals are used, but which do not meet the described conditions, are sharply distinguished from animal-assisted therapy. Examples of this are visiting services in homes, carried out by volunteers, or offerings such as hikes with llamas, visits to the farm, or courses with horses, led by people who are not professionals in animal-assisted therapy.[2]

Animal-assisted therapy should also not be confused with assistance by animals. So-called *assistance dogs* help and accompany people in everyday life. The best-known subgroup of assistance dogs are guide dogs for the blind, who help people with visual impairments to better manage their everyday life. Nowadays, there are numerous types of assistance dogs, which are either broadly positioned through their respective training or are specifically trained for one aspect. For example, there are diabetic alert dogs, seizure alert dogs, or asthma alert dogs, which are trained to signal or react in a certain way when the person is in an emergency situation due to a certain disease. There are also assistance dogs for mental illnesses or diseases with mental sequelae—such as dementia assistance dogs. The task of an assistance dog is to support the person as best as possible.

---

[2]The masculine form is used here and in the following and also for other designations (for example for patients, therapists etc.) for reasons of better readability and explicitly always includes both genders.

This support can look differently depending on the person's impairment. The assistance dog can either take over certain tasks that are difficult or impossible for the person, or it can react to a situation threatening to the person with early warning, or it can calm the person. In any case, an assistance dog has clear tasks and accompanies its person through everyday life.

A therapy support dog, on the other hand, does not accompany a specific person, but several patients. Moreover, its behavior is intended to help bring about a change in experience and behavior in the therapy participant as part of a therapy. Specifically, this means: The assistance dog is supposed to fulfill the wishes and needs of an impaired person; the therapy support dog, on the other hand, is supposed to encourage the patient to change their experience and behavior. So, the interaction with a therapy support dog is not about the dog performing certain exercises automatically. Instead, the therapeutic contact with the dog is about building and reflecting on relationships based on as free and unadulterated an encounter with the dog as possible.

▶ **Important!** A therapy support dog differs from an assistance dog. Therapy means change and thus development. The therapy support dog supports the development process within the framework of a therapy by initiating and accompanying a change process in the patient through its behavior and its effect. The developing relationship between human and therapy support dog offers the therapist many opportunities to invite the patient to reflect on relationships and to change interaction patterns. A therapeutically valuable relationship between patient and therapy support dog is therefore not hierarchical, but characterized by an encounter as free and unadulterated as possible.

When a dog is used in animal-assisted therapy, the dog is referred to as a *therapy support dog*. Sometimes, the misleading term "therapy dog" is used instead. The dog supports the therapy with its presence and behavior, but logically does not carry it out. It is rather the therapist who performs the therapy. Therefore, the correct designation for the dog is therapy *support* dog.

Also for animal-assisted therapy as a discipline, terms like "dog therapy" or "animal therapy" should be avoided. These terms are not only incorrect, but also misleading, as one could assume that the dog or the animal is being treated. As will be shown later, the term "Pet Therapy" which was frequently used in the past, is now outdated and no longer used. Today, only the term *animal-assisted therapy* is used. Variations and additions to this arise when a specific field of therapy is to be delimited or a specific form of therapy is meant, then for example, one speaks of animal-assisted occupational therapy.

1.2 Effective Factors and History of Animal-Assisted Therapy

"No person can give another the gift of idyll. Only an animal can do that" (Kundera,1988, p. 286).

As mentioned in the previous section, animals have always been present in almost all areas of human life. Considering this background, it is not surprising that animals are also used in human therapy. Nevertheless, this chapter serves to deepen the understanding of the reasons for using animals in therapy. Furthermore, the history of animal-assisted therapy as a discipline will be illuminated.

1.2.1 Effective Factors of Animal-Assisted Therapy—Why are Animals Good for Humans?

Much has been and is being speculated and researched about the exact factors that lead people to seek, appreciate, and benefit from contact with animals.

The so-called *Biophilia Hypothesis* is one of the more prominent theories. It was proposed in the mid-1980s by the sociobiologist Edward O. Wilson. Wilson defines biophilia as the human interest in animals in the sense of an "innate tendency to focus on life and lifelike processes" (Wilson quoted after Gullone, 2000, p. 293), that is, an inner striving of humans to focus on life itself and life-related processes. Wilson argues that in the development of humanity, it was a survival advantage for the individual human if he had the ability to assess the behavior of animals and find his way in nature. This has fundamentally shaped the human brain and human senses so that even in today's world—in which he usually no longer has to hunt, gather, and struggle for his survival in nature—he still has this strong inner connection to animals and nature.

In my opinion, the Biophilia Hypothesis explains well why humans feel connected to nature and observe and try to understand natural processes and animals with curiosity or interest. However, in my view, it falls short when it comes to explaining close, individual relationships between humans and animals. Why does a human build relationships with individual animals?

One approach to explaining human interest in dealing with animals, which focuses exactly on this aspect, puts the pronounced human desire for relationships in the spotlight and explains the special relationship between humans and animals from this perspective. The American family therapist Virginia Satir explains in the following words why contact with animals can be so beneficial for humans:

"Animals do not judge, they teach non-verbal (analog) communication, speak a "more honest" language, in which expression and what is meant correspond to each other. They speak the ancient language that our mother already spoke to us. It is the language of love, of grief, of struggle, of anger. It does not follow rules of syntax, logic, or grammar, but directly

expresses feelings for the other in an understandable way. It is the language of relationship."
(Satir quoted after Pottmann-Knapp, 2013, p. 5)

Satir, as mentioned, puts the relationship at the forefront of her explanations and names several reasons why humans can benefit from contact with animals and why animal-assisted therapy has thus emerged:

Firstly, the *unconditional acceptance,* which the human experiences through the animal. An animal does not judge by appearances, is not interested in a person's status in human society. Sometimes this aspect is also described as the *Cinderella effect*—through unconditional acceptance, the human can show his inner self and thus his true beauty in contact with the animal. Or to put it metaphorically: From the gray Cinderella, through the feeling of being accepted and appreciated, a proud princess emerges.

So instead of primarily reacting to appearances, an animal reacts to human behavior towards itself. For people who have experienced rejection or discrimination based on appearances, dealing with an animal can therefore be beneficial: the animal does not pay attention to appearances, but accepts the human as he is. And since every human in his life is confronted with human evaluation—perhaps also with prejudices—this unconditional acceptance by the animal is pleasant for most people:

> "Where a living being accepts us in our individual way, an emotional relationship begins that allows closeness and security, that opens us up to entrust ourselves emotionally to the other" (Otterstedt, 2001, pp. 34–35).

Another aspect that can make interaction with animals valuable for humans is the fact that we communicate with animals *analogously.* We humans can communicate both analogously or digitally. Analog communication is understood as communication through body language, facial expressions, and tone of voice. Digital communication, on the other hand, encompasses the content of spoken language. These two different forms of communication were described by psychotherapist and communication scientist Paul Watzlawick:

> "The difference between digital and analog communication becomes [clear] when one realizes that merely listening to an unknown language, e.g., on the radio, can never lead to understanding this language, while often quite extensive information can be relatively easily derived from the observation of sign languages and general expressive gestures, even if the person using them belongs to a foreign culture. Analog communication obviously has its roots in much more archaic periods of development and therefore has a much more general validity than the much younger and more abstract digital way of communication" (Watzlawick et al., 1974, pp. 62–63).

Communication with an animal, as is well known, does not take place through human language, but is always analog, as it happens on a bodily level—through touch, through eye contact, through the sound of the voice, through gestures and body tension.

This body-focused level of communication is, as Satir describes it, an "ancient language" (Satir quoted after Pottmann-Knapp, 2013, p. 5). Because before humans learn

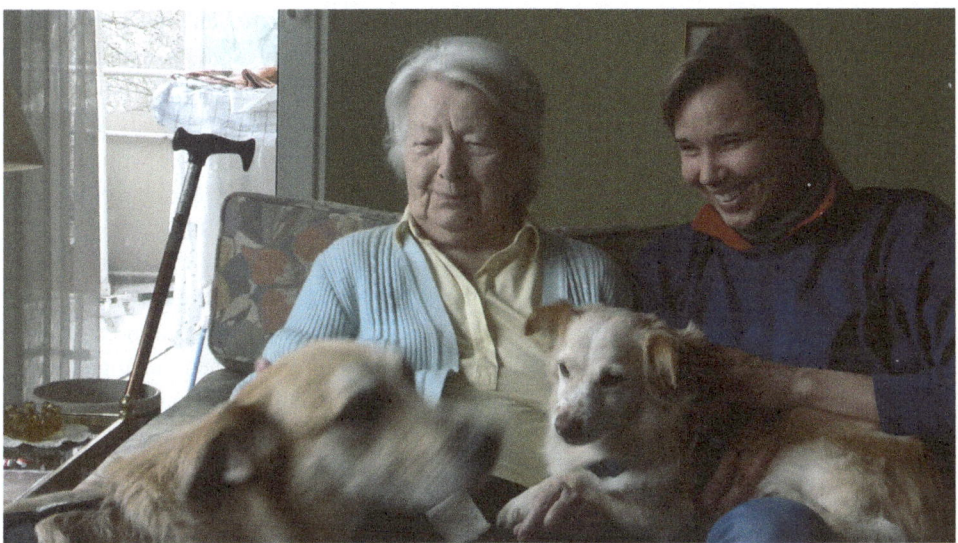

Fig. 1.1   Contact with the animal takes place on an emotional and relational level

actual speech, they communicate exclusively on this level, express their needs through it, receive feedback, comfort, and affection through it. The analog communication, which the animals in a way forces on us humans, thus directly touches the *feelings* of humans and brings them directly and *authentically* into relationship with the animal. This emotional and authentic communication with an animal conveys to humans *feelings of well-being and security*. Especially in contrast to situations that can occur and cause insecurity in human contact, such as when half-hearted statements are made or there is a contradiction between what is meant and what is said. These are so-called double messages, which can occur in human communication especially when digital and analog communication do not match.

In communication with the animal, however, such a contradiction cannot occur:

> "With animals, we speak analogously, and animals usually react promptly and clearly in body language to our communication behavior. With this, they fulfill two important factors for human learning and development: the immediacy of the reaction and the clarity of the reaction" (Olbrich et al., 2008, p. 55).

All of this leads to the fact that the healthy human—if he wants to engage and has not had bad experiences with animals—finds the encounter with an animal to be beneficial (see Fig. 1.1).

A person affected by physical or mental illness can particularly benefit from interacting with animals. The background to this is: Those who are ill usually also have to deal with *stress in the affective area* and changes or *difficulties in social relationships*. Mental illnesses almost always have a connection to the affective experience of the person, and physical illnesses also affect a person's emotional well-being. The same applies in this context to the relationships of the affected person, which can also be impaired by the mental or physical illness. Since interacting with animals directly appeals to human emotions and thus creates an authentic relationship with the animal, people with stress in the affective and social area generally find this interaction particularly enriching (Blesch, 2013; Otterstedt, 2001; Pottmann-Knapp, 2013; Proietti & La Gatta, 2005).

Or to put it another way: The more a person is impaired by his illness, the more important becomes to him the feeling of being accepted by someone else, and feeling comfortable and safe in contact with them. The previously described central aspects of contact with an animal—namely authenticity, unconditional acceptance, analogue communication, and emotional orientation—are therefore especially appreciated by people with physical or mental impairments.

1.2.2   Origins of Animal-Assisted Therapy

Animal-assisted therapy has only in recent decades been studied by scientists and become a popular term also to laypeople. However, initial approaches and attempts to help people through animal-assisted therapy can be traced back to the late eighteenth century. At that time, an English doctor, William Tuke, began encouraging his patients to care for animals. He worked in a psychiatric center sponsored by the Quakers and assumed that caring for weaker beings could improve his patients' impulse control. In the nineteenth century, an epilepsy center in Bielefeld, Germany, took a similar approach. A farm with horses and small animals was set up for the patients, and they were allowed to ride out and care for the animals. Another milestone in the history of animal-assisted therapy can be found in the twentieth century. In search of ways to rehabilitate soldiers traumatized by World War II, animals were also used for therapeutic purposes at the American "Pawling Army Air Force Convalescent Centre". Whether the fact that the psychoanalysts Sigmund Freud and C. G. Jung occasionally brought their dogs into therapy sessions (Pottmann-Knapp, 2013) is to be considered another stage or just a nice anecdote in this context is probably a matter of opinion.

The first real written representations of this therapy method emerged in the 1950s, and—in this context—the now outdated term *Pet Therapy*. American psychiatrist Boris Levinson noticed that a boy suffering from autism behaved more openly and he gained better access to him when Levinson's dog was in the practice. From then on, Levinson deliberately used his dog as a co-therapist in the boy's therapy and wrote the book "The dog as co-therapist", which coined the term Pet Therapy. Levinson's approach was taken up by the psychiatrist couple Corson in the 1970s and applied to the therapy of adults. Here the term *Pet Facilitated Therapy* was created. In the following decades, the still very isolated and special use of animals in therapy slowly expanded. Associations were formed, such as the American *Delta Society* (1977) or in the German-speaking area *Tiere helfen Menschen e.v.* (1987) and *Leben mit Tieren* (1988). First guidelines were issued and gradually training institutes, international networks like *IAHAIO* (= International Association of Human-Animal Interaction Organizations) and umbrella organizations like *ISAAT* (= International Society for Animal-Assisted Therapy) and *ESAAT* (= European Society for Animal-Assisted Therapy) were established.

Nowadays, however, the term Pet Therapy is no longer used, but instead we speak of *Animal-Assisted Therapy*. This term reflects the fact that the animal supports the therapy, but it is the therapist who carries out the therapy. Moreover, this term also describes the fact that not only classic pets are suitable for use in therapy, but also other domesticated animal species such as pigs, chickens or sheep.

In view of the growing seriousness and the demand for seriousness with which animal-assisted therapy is increasingly being carried out, there is now a stable endeavor to scientifically investigate and prove the effectiveness of animal-assisted therapy. Thus, there are now numerous studies on the effects of animal contact on human physical health:

As early as the 1980s, biologist Erika Friedmann investigated the influence of a pet on the survival probability of heart attack patients (Friedmann et al., 1980). It was found that patients with a pet had a higher survival probability than patients without a pet. It is worth noting that this effect remains even if dog owners are excluded, as they naturally move more. The authors therefore assume a stress-reducing effect of pets on humans and attribute the better health condition of pet owners in the study to this. This study was a milestone and at the same time a stimulus for further in-depth studies in the following years. It is proven, among other things, that:

- Pets have a higher stress-reducing influence on humans than the presence of a friend (Allen et al., 1991)
- a calming effect of a dog exists even when there is no direct physical contact between human and dog (ibid.)
- the presence of a dog lowers systolic and diastolic blood pressure and slows the pulse in people under mild stress, thereby calming them (ibid.)

Further studies clearly indicate a beneficial influence of animal-assisted therapy and activity on the human psyche. Studies have shown, among other things, that:

- Feelings of loneliness in nursing home residents are significantly reduced by the presence of an animal (Banks & Banks, 2002)
- Visits from therapy dogs can significantly increase the emotional well-being of cancer patients in treatment (The Mount Sinai Hospital, 2015)
- Anxiety in hospitalized patients significantly decreases through contact with animals (Barker & Dawson, 1998)

- Patients suffering from schizophrenia become more independent and competent in everyday life through animal-assisted therapy, and also develop a higher compliance towards therapy due to the bond with the animal (Kovács et al., 2004)
- Depressive symptoms of care-dependent people significantly reduce when they take care of an animal (Colombo et al., 2006)
- Animal-assisted activity influences the emotional states of nursing home residents more positively than music therapy activity (Blesch, 2013)

There are many other studies that could be listed, which have investigated the influence of animals and animal-assisted therapy on human mental and physical health in recent decades and years. The list provided here is therefore only to be understood as exemplary. A deeper insight into the research on animal-assisted therapy is provided by Pott-mann-Knapp, 2013; Beetz et al., 2018.

1.3   New Paths in Animal-Assisted Therapy

Animal-assisted therapy is a young and developing discipline. As previously described, a development towards more scientific rigor is taking place, which is to be welcomed for several reasons. Animal-assisted therapy is thus increasingly moving out of the niche area and becoming a serious therapeutic approach. In addition to deepening and expanding research on animal-assisted therapy, other developments must also take place. The establishment of binding training standards for professionals in animal-assisted therapy is one of such developments.

Another necessary development in animal-assisted therapy is the increase in interest and responsibility regarding issues of animal welfare and animal ethics.

For example, dolphin therapy, which emerged in the 70s, was considered for some time as an exciting and meaningful form of animal-assisted therapy until more and more concerns arose regarding animal welfare. Dolphins are wild animals, they do not live with humans, but are caught by humans and kept in aquariums to perform in shows or serve humans as "therapy animals". The capture of dolphins mostly takes place in brutal drive hunts by Japanese fishermen, who kill the dolphins for food purposes and at the same time catch some particularly beautiful dolphins alive to sell them to dolphinariums around the world. It is now known that about 50% of all captured dolphins do not survive the trauma of the drive hunt, the separation from their family, and the subsequent captivity (Kirsch, 2015). In 2014, a resolution against live captures of dolphins and whales was issued at the international species protection conference. It is undisputed that therapy with dolphins is against animal welfare and should no longer be carried out. Nevertheless, some countries like Turkey, Tunisia, or the USA still offer this animal welfare-violating and questionable form of therapy for a lot of money.

Dolphin therapy is an example of the need for further development in the sense of questioning common methods and views and opening up to the consideration of animal-assisted therapy from the perspective of the animals. We know that animal-assisted therapy can be beneficial to humans. Now it is important to include the perspective of the animals more strongly, to ask questions, to be open and curious, and to bring animal-assisted therapy onto new, more animal-friendly paths.

With the dog-assisted self-confidence training described in this book, I am trying to go new ways and to connect animal-assisted therapy and animal protection, or animal ethics. In this section, I would like to explain in more detail how this development came about by introducing my career path, my animal colleagues, and my conscious distancing from certain conservative views and explaining them.

1.3.1 My Professional Career

Since 2012, I have been working as a therapist at clinics for psychosomatics or psychiatry. During this time, I have designed the therapy concept with dogs presented in this book and continue to apply it to this day. The concept has slowly emerged, based on my previous experiences and training.

I am a graduate psychologist and have additional training in animal behavior therapy and a university education in animal-assisted therapy. Before starting my psychology studies, I studied philosophy and sociology for several semesters and during this time was a founding member and later chairwoman of the Animal Ethics Working Group at the University of Heidelberg. In preparing and conducting an interdisciplinary lecture series at the University of Heidelberg, I was able to meet renowned contemporary philosophers such as Tom Regan, Peter Wenz, or Eugen Drewermann and deal with animal ethical issues. Since I was primarily interested in the practical aspect, not least because of my experiences in animal protection collected in my youth, I then wanted to pursue a profession in which I could work with animals on the one hand and promote a positive human-animal relationship on the other.

I therefore decided to switch to psychology, specialized in my clinical internships in animal-assisted therapy, and completed my studies with field research on the effect of animal-assisted therapy on people in need of care. At the same time, I did additional training in animal behavior therapy and over time gained various practical experiences in animal-assisted work as well as in training dogs, horses (see Fig. 1.2) and cattle in Italy, Germany, Switzerland, Austria, and the USA. For several months each, I then worked in animal-assisted projects: first in an Italian center for riding and hippotherapy for multiply disabled children and adults, then in the Milan prison in an animal-assisted rehabilitation project with horses.

With the completion of the additional training in animal-assisted therapy at the Veterinary University of Vienna and in the context of my work as an individual and group therapist at a psychosomatic specialist clinic, I began to develop a concept for a dog-assisted group therapy (Blesch, 2015). Increasingly, I focused on animal-assisted individual therapies and gradually developed the dog-assisted self-confidence training. After

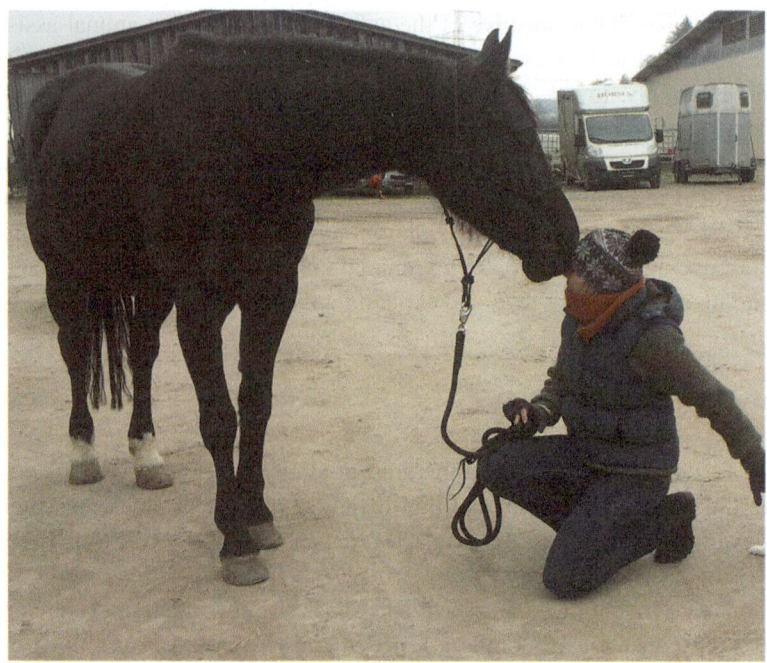

Fig. 1.2   My animal-assisted work began with horses—here with my current mare Marie

a change to another clinic, I specialized in this and work since then exclusively assisted by animals.

1.3.2   My Animal Colleagues

From the beginning of my activity, animal ethical convictions influenced my work. Therefore, all my animal colleagues come from animal protection. Currently, I work with rabbits, guinea pigs, and dogs. Since this book deals with animal-assisted work with dogs, they should be introduced in more detail at this point regarding their origin and their individual career paths:

Giulio has the most difficult past of my three dogs (see Fig. 1.3). Giulio is a shepherd mix and was probably born in 2007 in an Italian animal shelter. As a puppy, he was bitten by an older dog in the shelter, which led him to develop fear and mistrust towards his own kind. As a result, Giulio had to stay alone in his box. The years passed, and over time he developed physical ailments and behavioral disorders. He had chronic digestive problems and began to refuse food. He licked himself compulsively and shook the bars of his box so violently that he injured his canine teeth. The volunteers at the shelter urgently sought to find him a home, launching various appeals on the internet,

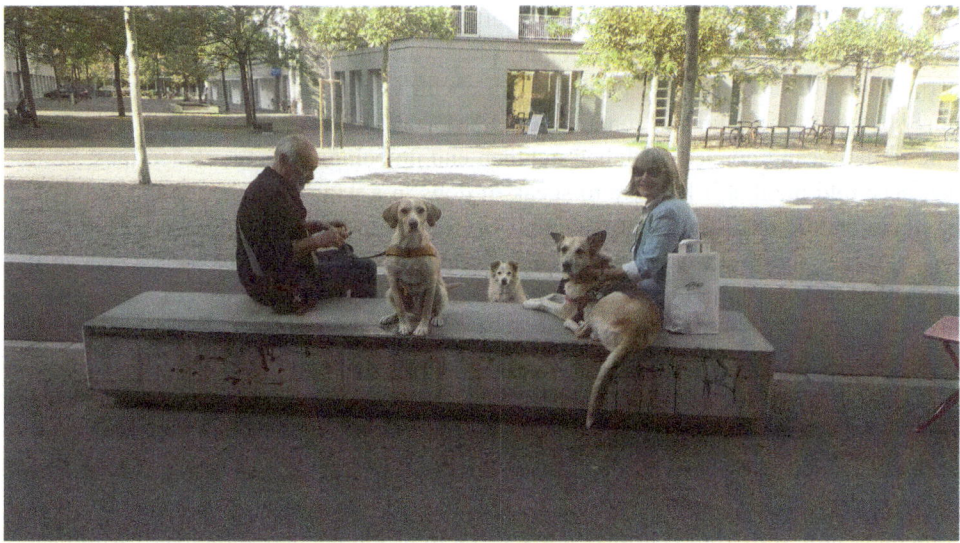

Fig. 1.3 Toni (left), Cleo, and Giulio with my parents

as they realized that Giulio, now about three years old, simply couldn't endure much longer in the kennel. That's how I found out about Giulio and got to know him. Despite some doubts, my family and I decided to take Giulio in. From the start, he was friendly and open towards us and our good-natured Golden Retriever, showing neither fear nor aggression, and was extremely in need of closeness and affection.

Training Giulio was not easy, as he had a lot of excess energy, showed hunting behavior, and was still afraid of strange dogs. It took several years, patience and understanding from all sides of the family, and a lot of training until Giulio became the dog he is now. Since 2012, he has been working at my side as a therapy companion dog. Giulio is the most sensitive and empathetic of all my dogs in dealing with the participants. He has been able to shed the shadows of his past, and so, beyond his concrete work with the participants, he functions in many therapies as a symbol of resilience and the always possible development and change in life—even when everything seems hopeless.

Cleo I adopted a few years after Giulio. She is a Spitz mix and a former street dog. She lived on the streets for many years, in a small pack consisting of her, her mother, and her brother. When all three fell seriously ill, they were captured. Her mother and brother died, but Cleo survived after a long, severe illness. Once fit again, she was taken to a shelter where she lived again in a small pack. Cleo is a survivor, self-confident, autonomous, and stubborn. And at the same time loyal, loving, and affectionate, once someone has won her favor.

While Giulio and Toni come running happily to greet a participant when they enter the door, Cleo initially stays relaxed and takes a good look at who is coming. If the person shows themselves to be friendly and self-confident, they can build a good and solid relationship with Cleo. Building a relationship with Cleo is therefore a process. Many participants therefore initially prefer to work with Giulio or Toni and only notice over time how much the calm and confident Cleo has to offer. There are not a few participants who initially can't connect with her and then end up being the biggest Cleo fans. Someone once told me that if he were to speak of dogs in a wine metaphor, then Cleo would be like a mature red wine while Toni and Giulio would be like a sparkling champagne. Even people who don't know wine can relate to champagne. An old red wine, on the other hand, is something for wine lovers. You have to engage with Cleo, she is something for dog connoisseurs and lovers.

Toni is the youngest of the three dogs in the pack. He too lived on the streets, but only for a few months, before he was caught by animal rights activists and brought to an animal shelter. That's where we brought him into the family. Toni is a hunting dog mix, energetic, intelligent, and enthusiastic about everything. If anyone always brings good vibes, it's Toni. He gets along with everyone and is very teachable. Practicing or training something new with Toni is always a joy, as he thinks along and participates with pleasure. Toni is also very adaptable. He is wilder and more playful with Giulio, but respectful and considerate with little Cleo. And he applies this sensitivity to the boundaries and needs of his counterpart to humans as well, reliably incorporating them into therapy.

On the one hand, I have introduced the dogs with whom I live and work in this section, as I could only develop and practice my animal-assisted concept thanks to them. On the other hand, the description of the dogs shows that I do not agree with all the common ideas about the practice of animal-assisted therapy. What I mean by that will be explained in the following section.

1.3.3   Delineation from Conservative Ideas in Animal-Assisted Therapy and Necessary Future Questions

There are four aspects of the previous or conservative way of understanding and applying animal-assisted therapy from which I consciously differentiate my work, namely the… :

- … too restrictive limitations regarding external factors of therapy companion animals
- … sometimes too pronounced curtailment of the natural expressions and behaviors of the animals
- … insufficiently formulated requirements for the species-appropriate handling of therapy companion animals
- … too few critical and fundamental questions concerning animal-assisted therapy as a discipline

In my understanding, the future of animal-assisted therapy lies, as mentioned, in questioning some of the previous ideas and opening up to animal ethical attitudes and new paths.

1.3.3.1 Focus on Behavior Rather than Appearances

The umbrella organization ESAAT, for example, requires that future therapy companion dogs have had "sufficient positive contact with humans, conspecifics and other animals and environmental stimuli" (ESAAT, p. 4) "already in the first two months of life". Although this requirement is something that every dog and every animal should be heartily wished for, it is not verifiable for dogs from animal welfare. If this requirement were actually applied, all dogs whose first eight weeks of life—for whatever reason—were not explicitly traceable, regardless of their behavior and character, would automatically be excluded from use as therapy companion dogs. And those who had to gather bad experiences, anyway. How many of the therapy companion dogs that have been faithfully, reliably, and successfully working for years, which I myself had and have or have met, would thus not be allowed to do their work! In my eyes, this regulation is obsolete and unnecessary. Because the suitability of a dog does not necessarily depend on this criterion. Instead, it depends on the *current behavior* and the *character* of the dog. I would like to explain this in more detail using the example of Giulio.

Throughout his service as a therapy dog, Giulio has worked with hundreds of participants.[3] At the end of the therapies, he was often bid farewell with tears, received countless farewell treats and thank you cards from participants. And this is because, through his loving, patient, and empathetic nature, he can provide a lot of comfort and at the same time, through his authentic reactions to the behavior of the participants, he provides valuable insights for the therapy of fundamental interactional difficulties.

Giulio is an excellent therapy dog. However, if one were to follow common conceptions, Giulio should never have been trained as a therapy dog. Because at the beginning of his development, he contradicted some rigid ideas about what a future therapy dog should be like. Instead of a puppy from controlled breeding of a popular dog breed, Giulio was a slightly over three-year-old mixed breed with a clear German Shepherd influence when he was adopted from the animal shelter. He had digestive problems and stress-related behavioral abnormalities. His puppyhood was characterized by fear of other dogs. As a puppy, young dog, and adult dog, he had hardly had the opportunity to have positive experiences with people, as he lived alone in a kennel between 23.5 and 24 hours a day and 365 days a year.

---

[3] I say "hundreds" because I can no longer count how many therapies Giulio has accompanied. As an individual and group therapist, in the first clinic where I worked with Giulio, I had twelve new patients every four to six weeks over a period of just over three years. Therefore, hundreds is a very modest estimate.

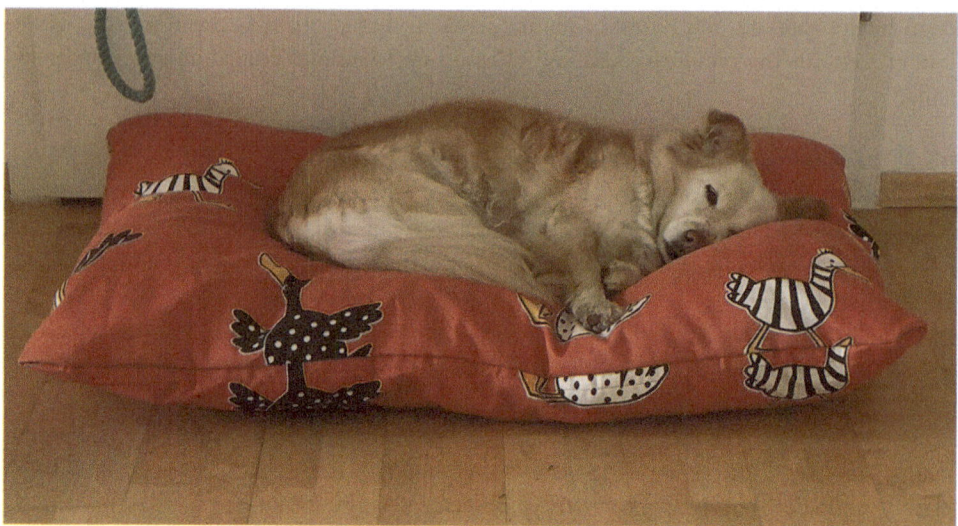

Fig. 1.4 Relaxed lying behavior on the side

So, at the beginning of his development, Giulio contradicted most of the rigid ideas about what a future therapy dog should be like: prepared for his future activity in puppy-hood, preferably belonging to a certain breed and coming from a breeder. Giulio was and is none of these, and yet he is the best therapy dog one could wish for.

And this is because in dog external criteria such as age, breed, or origin do not matter. Instead, what matters is his *behavior* and his *character*. Is the dog friendly and open towards people? Is he curious and open? Does he enjoy dealing with people? Is he kind and compatible? *These* are in my eyes the only important and meaningful criteria when it comes to assessing whether a dog is suitable for being trained as a therapy dog.

Since Giulio was all of this from the beginning, he was able to develop splendidly with the help of the necessary training. He has been able to shed his fears of other dogs with few exceptions and has now lived for many years as a proud pack leader with Cleo and Toni as well as with the previous other family dogs. He eats with the great appetite that is typically inherent in most dogs, has no physical complaints, only has to go to the vet for vaccinations and check-ups. He no longer shows any stereotypical behavioral abnormalities and has a reliable and balanced nature.

So, dogs from animal welfare can become just as good therapy dogs as dogs from breeders. This is the first and most important distinction between my way of planning and conducting animal-assisted therapy and common conceptions.

1.3.3.2 Allowing Authenticity Instead of Curtailing Natural Expressions

As previously described, there are now countless institutes and private individuals who offer courses and training in animal-assisted therapy (see Sect. 1.2.2). In some of the associated examination regulations or statutes, which set out the requirements for the therapy dog, certain expectations of the dog's behavior are listed that I do not entirely share.

Without wanting to single out individual institutes or persons, one can repeatedly find, for example, the following requirement for the therapy dog: The dog must be able to lie down without problems at the feet or next to a person unfamiliar to the dog. This is something I do not expect from my dogs—on the contrary.

Indeed, it can be very revealing under certain circumstances to let the dog decide where and how it wants to lie down. A dog expresses various things through the way it lies and the proximity or distance it maintains. If it lies on its side, openly showing its belly, with its head laid to the side, well, then we know: it is relaxed and feels comfortable with the people in its environment (see Fig. 1.4). If it lies propped up on its paws, with its head upright, the dog is in a kind of waiting position. It may be that it is actually waiting for something. But it could also be that it perceives a certain tension from the people around it, cannot fully relax in the situation and therefore assumes this position, in which it is ready to get up and act. *How* the dog lies during therapy thus shows us how it assesses the situation and the people around it and what state it is in as a result.

Where the dog lies is also revealing. Does it lie in close proximity to the participant? Perhaps even on the floor directly at their feet? Does it seek physical contact while lying down? Does it lie down in its resting place? Does it lie down next to the therapist?

The proximity that the dog *voluntarily* takes to the participant indicates how close it *wants* to be to the participant. A dog can hardly express its feelings in relation to the participant more clearly.

So I would never dictate to my dogs where and how they should lie down in therapy so that the patient can, for example, pet them well.[4] Not only because I want to respect my dogs' personal boundaries. But also and especially because I would take away a lot from the therapy process by doing so.

Example: Spontaneous lying behavior of the dog as important input for therapy

A participant with a complex personality structure, who suffers from relationship conflicts with various people in her everyday life, comes to animal-assisted therapy to strengthen her self-esteem. In the interaction with Giulio, this participant initially sends contradictory messages. For example, she talks to Giulio at the beginning of the session, but as soon as he comes to her and offers contact, she turns away from him again. He stays next to her for a while, waiting to see if she might still want to pet him, but when no further reaction from her occurs, he lies down on his resting

---

[4]There is certainly a difference when dogs are used as visiting dogs for seriously ill people. A visiting dog for a person in a coma or for a person bedridden for other reasons has different tasks than a therapy companion dog used in the therapy of people with mental illnesses.

place. As soon as he lies there, the participant addresses him again, but Giulio remains lying away from her. The participant expresses disappointment and sadness that Giulio has moved away from her and does not come to her despite being addressed. She feels confirmed in her low self-esteem.

This reaction of the participant to Giulio's lying behavior becomes the starting point for addressing and working on the participant's fundamental behavioral patterns. The participant initially only feels the disappointment about Giulio's distant lying and devalues herself as a person. She does not yet recognize that it is not her person, but her behavior that is causally responsible for Giulio's lying behavior. Talking to him, but neither looking at him nor touching him when he comes to her, these are contradictory messages for Giulio. Giulio cannot assess her behavior, does not know whether she wants closeness to him or not, and therefore initially keeps his distance from her. He does not reject her as a person, but cannot interpret her behavior and therefore becomes insecure and keeps his distance. In the discussion about the relationship dynamics between the participant and Giulio, it becomes clear that similar dynamics exist in her interpersonal relationships. Unclear messages regarding closeness and distance, distancing due to insecurity, disappointment, accusations, self-doubt—these are some of the participant's experience and behavior patterns in her relationships that become apparent later on.

Through what Giulio's spontaneous lying behavior triggered in the participant and the analysis of the reasons for this lying behavior, we thus gained access to the core of the participant's interactional difficulties. ◀

As the example shows, the dog's lying behavior is an expression of his immediate feeling and his assessment of the participant. Dogs are very sensitive to contradictory messages, react immediately to them, and express their reaction through their spontaneous behavior—for example, as Giulio did with his distance behavior.

So, I encourage the authentic behaviors and natural expressions of my dogs, rather than curtailing them, as is done in some training. The lying behavior serves as a tangible example because, in my view, it clearly shows the importance of allowing spontaneous behaviors of the dog. But it also applies to other behaviors. My dogs are allowed to lie down wherever they want, they are allowed to move freely in the room,—in short: they are allowed to express their feelings freely at any time. Only this circumstance offers me the opportunity to work therapeutically. Because the behavior of the dogs reflects the behavior of the participant. The behavior of the dogs makes the behavior of the participant visible to me, thereby making it discussable and ultimately changeable.

▶   **Important!** Only by allowing the dog's natural behaviors is it possible to work therapeutically. The dog's spontaneous reactions reflect the behavior of the participant. This can make fundamental behavioral patterns of the participant visible to the therapist. The therapist can then address these, question the participant's interpersonal relationships in this regard, and initiate change processes.

I would like to emphasize at this point the obvious fact that, despite all the behavioral freedom granted, I do not allow aggressive behavior from the dogs. As described later, I ensure during the selection of the dog that it does not show any aggressive behavior towards humans (see Sects. 4.1 and 4.2). The dogs are thus free in their authentic expression within the limits of good interaction with each other.

1.3.3.3 More Rules for Providers

Another point of criticism I have about the current state of animal-assisted therapy is that too few rules are imposed on providers in their interaction with the animals.

The frequency of an animal's use, the duration of a therapy unit, the content design of a session, and the creation of necessary balance are left to the respective professional. There are, if any, isolated recommendations, but without claiming to be binding. This may also be due to the fact that animals differ in some needs and every therapy environment is different. This makes it difficult to establish universally applicable rules. What is specifically missing, however, is that animal-assisted therapy as a discipline asks fundamental questions about its interaction with animals and its concept of the human-animal relationship. And that these questions are seriously, scientifically based and worked on in exchange with other disciplines.

Thus, the difficulty of too few binding rules for providers only resolves when animal-assisted therapy begins to ask general questions concerning the animals.

1.3.3.4 Inclusion of Animal Ethics

Animal-assisted therapy emerged as a discipline because initially individual therapists and over the decades also the general public noticed that contact with animals is beneficial to humans. In an effort to gain recognition as a form of therapy, scientific studies were conducted based on this and today there is ample evidence for the effectiveness of animal-assisted therapy. There are various attempts and approaches to work with animals in almost all therapeutic areas in the broadest sense: from animal-assisted dentistry (to alleviate fears of dentist visits through the presence of an animal) to animal-assisted pelvic floor training for pregnant women to animal-assisted nature education. With the additional designation "animal-assisted" almost everything imaginable exists.

However, if the discipline wants to establish itself seriously, it must evolve and build a future perspective. Just "carry on" and occupy as many, sometimes exotic, fringe areas of therapy as possible, that is, in my view, the wrong way. Because especially in today's times, in which we are directly experiencing the consequences of human exploitation of nature and its resources, more and more people are questioning the self-evidence with which decisions are made about nature and animals without including their perspective. This self-evidence, with which we humans assume to have the right to decide about animals and their lives, is impressively illustrated by the writer Milan Kundera several decades ago with the following words:

> "At the beginning of Genesis it is written that God created man to rule over fowl, fish, and beast. However, Genesis was written by a man, not a horse. There is no certainty that God actually entrusted man with dominion over other creatures. It is much more likely that man invented God to sanctify the dominion he has seized over cow and horse. Indeed, the right to kill a deer or a cow is the only thing that all of humanity unanimously agrees on, even during the bloodiest wars. This right seems self-evident to us because we are at the top of the hierarchy. But all it would take is for a third party to enter the game, such as a visitor from another planet, whose God would have said: 'You will rule over the creatures of the other stars', and suddenly the self-evidence of Genesis would become problematic. The man who is harnessed to a cart by a Martian or roasted on a spit by a resident of the Milky Way, may perhaps remember the veal cutlet he was used to cutting on his plate, and he will apologize (too late!) to the cow." (Kundera, 1988, pp. 273–274).

Animal Protection Law versus Animal Ethics

The Animal Protection Law is intended to protect animals from arbitrariness. Thus, at the beginning of the law, it states:

> "The purpose of this law is to protect the life and well-being of animals as fellow creatures from the responsibility of humans. No one may inflict pain, suffering or harm on an animal without reasonable cause" (German Animal Protection Law, § 1).

This approach is initially to be valued as positive, yet the addition of "without reasonable cause" includes a huge scope for humans. If something benefits humans, a "reasonable cause" is quickly found. The Animal Protection Law may punish sadistic actions and slightly reduce torturous forms of keeping by formulating certain minimum standards, but ultimately the interest of humans is always in the foreground. The Animal Protection Law does not ask what is *morally right* in dealing with animals.

Animal ethics, on the other hand, asks exactly this question. It asks what interests animals have—and initially regardless of whether these are compatible with human interests. Animal ethics is about the animal and the moral relationship to humans—and this clearly, comprehensively, and soberly.

In today's age, in which people are increasingly called upon to question themselves, their actions, and their impact, it is crucial for the field of animal-assisted therapy to seriously and openly include the perspective of the animals involved. Too little has been asked so far:

- Contact with animals is good for humans, but what about the animal?
- Is the animal's involvement beneficial for it?
- What conditions must be considered for an animal's involvement to be beneficial?
- Do we need to consider the interests of the animals?
- If so, how do we recognize the interests of the animal?

- And fundamentally: *Are* we humans ethically allowed to use animals as therapy companions without a second thought?
- And the underlying question is: Is a sentient being with its own interests and needs allowed to serve as a *means to an end*?

Animal-assisted therapy should start asking these questions. For too long, the impact of animal-assisted therapy on the animals and the fundamental question of whether it is even animal-friendly to use an animal for therapeutic purposes have been simply ignored. It's about taking the animals and their concerns seriously—beyond a superficial commitment to minimum animal welfare standards or general animal protection laws. And it is *animal ethics* that, as almost the only field, *seriously places the concerns of animals at the center*. Therefore, dealing with the questions and answers of animal ethics is necessary and forward-looking for the further development of animal-assisted therapy.

References

Allen, K. M., Blascovich, J., Tomaka, J., & Kelsey, R. M. (1991). Presence of human friends and pet dogs as moderators of autonomic respondes to stress in women. *Journal of Personality and Social Psychology, 61*(4), 582–589.

Banks, M. R., & Banks, W. A. (2002). The effects of animal-assisted therapy on loneliness in an elderly population in long-term care facilities. *Journal of Gerontology, 57A*(7), 428–432.

Barker, S. B., & Dawson, K. S. (1998). The effects of animal-assisted therapy on anxiety ratings of hospitalized psychiatric patients. *Psychiatric Services, 49*(6), 797–801.

Beetz, A., Riedel, M., & Wohlfarth, R. (Eds.). (2018). *Tiergestützte Interventionen: Handbuch für Aus- und Weiterbildung*. Ernst Reinhardt.

Blesch, K. (2013). *Hunde—Musik—Emotionen. Ein empirischer Vergleich der Wirkung von tiergestützter und musiktherapeutischer Aktivität*. AV Akademiker.

Blesch, K. (2015). Tiergestützte Gruppenpsychotherapie. *Gruppenpsychotherapie—Gruppendynamik, 51*, 86–97.

Colombo, G., Dello Buono, M., Smania, K., Raviola, R., & De Leo, D. (2006). Pet Therapy and institutionalized elderly: A study on 144 cognitively unimpaired subjects. *Archives of Gerontology and Geriatrics, 42*, 207–216.

ESAAT. (2012). Definition tiergestützter Therapie. https://www.esaat.org/definition-tiergestuetzter-therapie/. Accessed: 18. Dec. 2019.

Friedmann, E., Katcher, A. H., Lynch, J. J., & Thomas, S. A. (1980). Animal companions and one-year survival of patients after discharge froma coronary care unit. *Public Health Report, 95*, 307–312.

Gullone, E. (2000). The biophilia hyothesis and life in the 21st century: Increasing mental health or increasing pathology? *Journal of Happiness Studes, 1*(3), 293–322.

Kirsch, U. (2015). Delfintherapie—Geschäftemacherei auf Kosten der Patienten und der Delfine. https://www.delphinschutz.org/delfine/delfintherapie/. Accessed: 3. Jan. 2020.

Kovács, Z., Kis, R., Rózsa, S., & Rózsa, L. (2004). Animal-assisted therapy for middle-aged schizophrenic patients living in a social institution. A pilot study. *Clinical Rehabilitation, 18*, 483–486.

Kundera, M. (1988). *Die unerträgliche Leichtigkeit des Seins*. Fischer Taschenbuch.

Olbrich, E., Beetz, A., & Julius, H. (2008). Elemente einer Theorie der Mensch-Tier-Beziehung. In Grosse-Siestrup et al. (Eds.), *Kongress Mensch und Tier—Tiere in der Prävention und Therapie 2008* (p. 160). http://www.mensch-tier-kongress.de.

Otterstedt, C. (2001). *Tiere als therapeutische Begleiter*. Kosmos.

Pottmann-Knapp, B. (2013). *Tiergestützte (Psycho)Therapie—Wissen für Diagnostik, Behandlung, Therapie, Prävention, Salutogenese, Resilienz, Förderung, Entwicklung, Begleitung*. AV Akademiker.

Proietti, G., & La Gatta, W. (2005). *La Pet Therapy*. Xenia Edizioni.

Seeberg, U. (2008). Das Bild des Tieres in der Höhlenmalerei. In J. Ullrich, F. Weltzien & H. Fuhlbrügge (Eds.), *Ich, das Tier*. Dietrich Reimer.

The Mount Sinai Hospital. (13. Januar 2015). Clinical trial shows benefit of animal-assisted therapy in adult cancer patients undergoing complex cancer treatment with chemotherapy, radiation therapy. *ScienceDaily*. www.sciencedaily.com/releases/2015/01/0150113154029.htm. Accessed: 18. Dec. 2019

Watzlawick, P., Beavin, J. H., & Jackson, D. D. (1974). *Menschliche Kommunikation—Formen, Störungen, Paradoxien*. Hans Huber.

Animal Ethics in Animal-Assisted Therapy

2

Contents

Abstract

This chapter deals with animal ethics and thus with socially significant, current questions regarding human interaction with animals. The first part is about understanding why important questions about ethically correct behavior towards animals have so far received little attention in animal-assisted therapy. Subsequently, animal ethics are presented in a summarized and abbreviated form. The focus here is on the most well-known representatives and currents of animal ethics. The chapter finally culminates in the question relevant for the future development of animal-assisted therapy, what questions and ethical obligations animal ethics gives us as animal-assisted therapists.

K. Blesch, *Animal-Assisted Therapy with Dogs*,
https://doi.org/10.1007/978-3-662-67965-4_2

2.1   Lack of Consideration of Animal Ethical Issues in Animal-Assisted Therapy

Both animal ethics and animal-assisted therapy deal with the human-animal relationship. However, so far, both disciplines have hardly referred to each other. How come?

Firstly, it should be noted that the human-animal relationship is complex, multifaceted, and contradictory. On the one hand, the situation of cows, pigs, chickens, and other so-called "livestock" is worsening due to the steadily increasing consumption of animal products and the advancing mechanization of rearing and killing. On the other hand, humans are increasingly living with so-called "pets", caring for them better and better, so that they live longer and healthier on average. Or to put it in numbers: In Germany, 750 million animals are killed annually for food production (Animal Equality Germany e. V., 2019), with 99% of these animals coming from factory farming (ibid.). At the same time, the number of pets in Germany is steadily increasing—by about 3.8 million to around 34.4 million pets between 2016 and 2018 alone (Statista, 2019). This boundary drawn by humans between the categories of livestock and pets appears all the more arbitrary when one considers that it has been scientifically proven for years that, for example:

- Pigs perform better in intelligence tests than dogs (Hatkoff, 2009, p. 97),
- Chickens possess object permanence from hatching—a skill that human infants only develop between the ages of five and eight months (ibid., p. 22),
- Cattle can not only solve problems, but react joyfully and enthusiastically to their success, which is an important indicator of self-awareness (ibid., p. 62).

Especially in view of the ambivalence with which humans deal with different animal species, one would assume that there would be a lively exchange between the different disciplines dealing with the human-animal relationship, and that animal ethical issues would be discussed in all animal-relevant disciplines. Unfortunately, the reality is completely different: animal-assisted therapy, as one of the central disciplines in the field of human-animal relationships, has so far paid little or no attention to the basic findings of animal ethics.

The reason for this is quite simple: Animal ethics, based in philosophy, raises fundamental questions about how we deal with animals—and this *regardless* of whether a particular interaction with an animal is pleasant or useful to humans. Instead of asking: What is good for humans?, animal ethics asks: What is *the ethically right* thing to do? Animal-assisted therapy, which aims to increase human well-being through the use of animals, can therefore easily be put under pressure by some, perhaps ruthless, questions of animal ethics. Because so far, it is (still) the absolute exception in animal-assisted therapy that the interests of the animals are given the same weight as the interests of the human patients or clients. For example, therapy animals are granted rest periods between therapy units, but it is still rarely critically questioned:

- whether it is right that the conventional training of an animal for use in therapy includes the suppression of certain natural expressions,
- whether the animal enjoys the therapy as much as the patient does,
- or whether the therapy is good for the animal in the short and long term.

Therefore, it is primarily the animal-assisted therapists who avoid engaging with animal ethics and information and questions from this area. The underlying fear is often that a critical examination of individual aspects could completely question their own activity (and thus perhaps their own basis for existence). American Professor of Social Psychology Melanie Joy refers to this as the phenomenon of *confirmation bias* or *Tolstoy Syndrome*.[1]

> "Most people, even the most intelligent, [have] trouble recognizing the truth—even the simplest and clearest truth, if this truth forces them to consider ideas they have based their lives on as wrong." (Joy, 2013, p. 150).

The avoidance of dealing with animal ethics is therefore not due to a lack of interest or even ill will. It usually happens for self-protection. While such avoidance may be understandable, it still represents a serious omission. It is undisputed that psychologists, psychotherapists, doctors, physiotherapists or occupational therapists must have and practice an ethically correct view of humanity in order to carry out their activities. Why should anything different apply to animal-assisted therapists? Since the animal-assisted therapist works with both humans *and* animals, every practitioner in this field must openly and critically engage with their attitude towards animals and their image of the human-animal relationship. Only in this way can they work seriously in today's complex field of tension in the human-animal relationship. And animal-assisted therapy as a discipline must deal with its neighboring disciplines, ask itself critical questions, allow insights and possibly further develop them and adapt its own actions accordingly. Otherwise, the further development of the field is not possible. The discussion of animal ethical questions is therefore a challenge aimed at the future of animal-assisted therapy, which the field and every individual therapist must face.

In the following, I will first summarize the most important positions of animal ethics in order to then relate the questions and insights of animal ethics to animal-assisted work and to ask the decisive question from an animal ethical point of view: Is animal-assisted therapy ethically justifiable?

---

[1] This phenomenon was named after the writer Tolstoy, as he described how difficult it can be to convey a simple truth based on facts to someone who is already convinced of the opposite.

Summary: Previous Handling of Animal Ethics in Animal-Assisted Therapy

Both animal ethics and animal-assisted therapy deal with the human-animal relationship. However, there is currently too little exchange between the two disciplines. It is primarily the animal-assisted therapists who often still avoid dealing with animal ethics. In the background, there is often the fear that animal ethics raises critical questions that could completely question the use of animals in human therapy. A rethinking in the sense of shedding this fear and thus opening up to questions from animal ethics is necessary for the further development of animal-assisted therapy.

2.2   Animal Ethics

Animal ethics examines and analyzes the ethical questions associated with human relationships, human behavior, and human views on animals.

▶ **Definition "Ethics" and "Animal Ethics"** "Ethics is the systematic study of the question of good and bad human action. […] According to [this] understanding, animal ethics is therefore the systematic study of the question of how we should behave towards non-human animals, and the formulation of reasoned answers to this question." (Blesch et al., 2007, p. 5)

The ethics of human action towards animals has been repeatedly presented as an elementary character test by various thinkers. Kundera formulates it as follows:

> "True human goodness, in its absolute purity and freedom, can only manifest itself to those who represent no power. The true moral test of humanity, the elementary test (…) is expressed in the relationship of humans to those who are at their mercy: to the animals" (Kundera, 1988, p. 277).

There are also other lines of thought and positions on the ethical duties of humans towards animals (see Sect. 2.2.1). Thus, over the past decades and centuries, those philosophers and scientists who have dealt with this question of the right action towards animals have given different answers based on different justifications. Animal ethics has now become a very complex discipline of philosophical ethics. This complexity is also due to overlaps with other disciplines such as neuroscience or behavioral biology and their influences on the animal ethics discourse. New insights about animal behavior or animal perception and pain sensitivity change the discourse or bring new aspects into the discussion. Considering this, I can and want to give only a general overview of animal ethics at this point and at the same time refer to the most important works on the subject for a deeper examination.

2.2.1   Anthropocentrism

In animal ethics, there are philosophers like the contemporary representative Carl Cohen, who provide a theoretical framework for the implicit attitude of most people, namely: animals should not be tortured without reason, but they have no rights because they are not part of the human moral community:

> "Humans have many duties towards animals—few will dispute that. But it certainly does not follow that animals have rights" (Cohen quoted by Blesch et al., 2007, p. 94).

Such an answer to the question of the correct human behavior towards animals we call *ethical anthropocentrism*. The lines of argumentation prove to be quite fragile upon closer examination. Because in the discussions, so-called exclusion criteria are argued. These are certain facts (or assumptions) which underline the difference between humans and animals and argue that humans have no moral duties towards animals. A possible argument with exclusion criterion would be: animals have no rights because they themselves cannot make moral decisions, or animals have no rights because they are less intelligent than humans. The ability to make moral decisions or intelligence are in this case the exclusion criteria, the reasons why a boundary is drawn between two groups.

Against many of these exclusion criteria, valid counterarguments can be found. If we take intelligence as an exclusion criterion, for example, the parrot, which has the intelligence quotient of a toddler, puts us in an argumentative predicament. If we refer to the ability to act morally, toddlers and people with certain mental disabilities put us in distress. In short: as a rule, the arguments that we use as exclusion criteria are relativized by certain members of the human species or by certain highly developed non-human species and thus refuted in their universality. The only line of argument left is: humans have rights because they are humans, and all other animal species have no rights because they are not humans. The subjectivity and circularity of this argument becomes clear when we replace the terms and say, for example: rabbits have rights because they are rabbits, and all other animal species have no rights because they are not rabbits. We argue here exclusively from the assumption of the primacy of our own species—from a logical and ethical point of view, a rather subjective and incorrect approach (see *speciesism* Sect. 2.2.2).

A common phenomenon within anthropocentrism is not only the separation between humans and other animal species, but also the discrepancy described at the beginning (Sect. 2.1), by which different animal species are treated. As social psychologist Melanie Joy describes it:

> "We do not love dogs for the reason and do not eat cows for the reason because dogs and cows would be fundamentally different—cows have feelings, preferences, and a consciousness just like dogs—but because we *perceive* them as different" (Joy, 2013, p. 14)

Joy attributes this perception to an implicit, culturally conditioned schema (she refers to this as *carnism*), according to which humans classify animals as edible or non-edible.

This classification of animals is followed by a perception process that determines our actions. Specifically: most members of the Western cultural circle would feel disgust (= perception) and react with rejection (= action) if they were offered the meat of a Golden Retriever puppy. At the same time, however, eating a veal fillet is considered normal and natural. Thus, humans culturally classify different animal species into categories. This categorization then determines what we feel for these animal species—whether we feel disgust at the thought of eating them, whether we have compassion for them, whether we grant them the right to life. Joy thus provides an explanation for the ambivalence of the human relationship to different animal species with her concept of carnism and at the same time advocates a change in the arbitrary classification of animals into utility or pets. The keys to this include:

- The *critical questioning* of the correctness of our categorization system
- The *"reification" of so-called farm animals*, in which a cow is perceived as what it is, namely not as a soulless object, but as an individual with desires, goals, and a memory
- The *development of empathy* for animals in general—including animals that we do not classify as pets

Summary: The Red Lines of Anthropocentrism
Speciesism (see Sect. 2.2.2)
    In anthropocentrism, a red line is drawn between the human species and other animal species—without this being justifiable by "hard facts" (i.e., actual differences affecting all members of a species in anatomy, intelligence, behavior, perception, or emotions).
    Carnism (see Sect. 2.2.1)
    In anthropocentrism, a further red line is drawn between so-called pets and farm animals. This is also not justifiable by "hard facts".

2.2.2 Non-Anthropocentrism

The counter-position to anthropocentrism is *non-anthropocentrism*. This umbrella term encompasses those currents of animal ethics that assume that not only humans are part of the moral community, but that other sentient beings are also to be considered. I will introduce the two main currents of animal ethics, namely *teleological* and *deontological ethics,* in the following.

    The *teleological approach*[2] is primarily interested in the pursued purpose, or the ultimately achieved goal, when ethically evaluating an action. An example of the teleologi-

---

[2] Derived from the Greek term *télos* for "the purpose" and/or "the goal".

cal approach is the most frequently discussed *preference utilitarianism* according to the Australian philosopher Peter Singer, the founder of modern animal ethics. Singer was one of the first modern philosophers to put the discourse on animal rights at the center, did so clearly and distinctly, and was criticized just as clearly and distinctly.

According to Singer, the basis of an ethical decision is a cost-benefit analysis that satisfies the most interests. Here, the interests of animals are explicitly included and are equivalent to human interests:

> "I believe that our current attitude towards [non-human animals] is based on a long history of prejudice and arbitrary discrimination. I assert that there can be no reason—apart from the selfish striving of the exploiting group to preserve their privileges—to deny the extension of the basic principle of equal consideration to members of other species" (Singer, 1996, p. 12).

The starting assumption for including the interests of animals for Singer is thus the *principle of equality*—that is, the assumption that one's own interests or the interests of the group to which someone feels they belong have the same weight as the interests of persons or beings who are different from us. The principle of equality is the moral argument against racism, against sexism, and—since Singer—against *speciesism*, i.e., against the "attitude of bias in favor of the interests of members of one's own species" (Singer, 1996, p. 35). Singer also refers to the English philosopher, thinker, and reformer Jeremy Bentham, born over 250 years ago, whose optimistic view of the future describes the attitude of many of today's animal ethicists with the following words:

> "The day will come when the rest of the living creatures will be granted the rights that could only be withheld from them by tyranny. The French have already recognized that the blackness of the skin is no reason to leave a human being defenseless to the whims of a tormentor. One day it will be recognized that the number of legs, the hairiness of the skin, and the end of the os sacrum are all insufficient reasons to leave a sentient being to the same fate. But what other characteristic could be the insurmountable boundary? [...] The question is not: Can they *think*? or: Can they *speak*?, but: Can they *suffer*?" (Bentham quoted after Singer, 1996, pp. 35–36).

However, since utilitarianism is about weighing interests, the inclusion of animal interests explicitly does not mean that killing animals or causing them suffering would be ethically forbidden per se. Thus, a prohibition on killing presupposes that the animal has the ability for self-awareness and a concept of the future. Only then can an interest in continuing to live be established. These abilities are attributed to animal species with intelligence similar to human intelligence, such as primates. Apart from that, it is a matter of weighing interests. If the suffering of animals caused by a human action is greater than the benefit to humans, this action should be rejected.

Parallel to utilitarianism as part of teleological ethics, there exists in animal ethics, as mentioned above, the *deontological approach*.[3] This focuses on the inner motives, principles of action, and duties in the ethical consideration of an action. It asks whether ethical basic principles are followed in a decision. This is not about a cost-benefit analysis as in utilitarianism, but philosophers of this direction ask about the individual and their decision for a certain action or behavior. This current in animal ethics follows the philosophy of the founder of the Enlightenment, Immanuel Kant. He assumed that humans as rational and autonomous beings represent a purpose in themselves, and thus, regardless of advantages or disadvantages, there is always a moral duty to treat them with respect. The prevailing worldview and the associated ideas about humans and animals began to slowly change:

Excursus: Capacity to suffer—an important term in animal ethics
The capacity to suffer is the ability of a living being to experience suffering. It is closely linked to the discussion about pain perception and consciousness. The aspect of the capacity to suffer is used by many philosophers and other scientists as a decisive criterion when it comes to which ethical principles should apply in dealing with a species. The difficulty is: "Suffering cannot be measured with scientific methods" (Würbel in Blesch et al., 2007, p. 19).

Nevertheless, animals were long simply denied the ability to suffer. This happened on the basis of the Cartesian worldview, in which non-human animals were considered objects without consciousness.

Since animals cannot communicate in our language and we cannot directly measure the ability to suffer, other approaches are needed. A conclusive approach to clarify whether an animal is capable of suffering, or is suffering, is the so-called *analogy conclusion* between humans and animals:

> "Accordingly, we can conclude that an animal is suffering if the animal (1) has a nervous system that is anatomically and physiologically similar to humans, (2) is exposed to a situation that is comparable to a situation that would cause suffering in us humans, and (3) simultaneously shows reactions (physiological and in behavior) that are comparable to those that we humans would show in a comparable situation and with corresponding suffering" (ibid., p. 19).

This analogy conclusion does not mean that the ability to suffer does not also exist in animals that resemble humans less strongly or not at all. This approach is an opening and a beginning to recognize other living beings than humans as capable of suffering and thus as capable of feeling and consciousness.

---

[3] Derived from the Greek term *deon* for "the obligatory".

"After overcoming the Cartesian worldview, which particularly emphasized humans as rationally gifted beings, the general appreciation of morality in the 18th century led to the recognition of the ability to suffer and feel as a moral criterion" (Goetschel and Bolliger in Blesch et al., 2007, p. 179).

While Kant referred exclusively to humans and excluded animals as members of the moral community, the philosopher Arthur Schopenhauer in the nineteenth century extended Kantian ethics. Schopenhauer criticized the attitude of drawing a sharp distinction between humans and animals in terms of their ability to suffer. And so, within the framework of his *compassion ethics*, Schopenhauer extended human morality to the treatment of animals. While Kant based his ethical considerations only on *rational* beings, i.e., humans, Schopenhauer explicitly included all *sentient* beings, i.e., animals, in his compassion ethics.

A similar attitude is found in the philosopher and physician Albert Schweitzer, who speaks of a unity of all living beings and thus a necessary reverence of man for life itself and thus also for animals:

"I call upon humanity to the ethics of reverence for life. This ethic makes no distinction between more valuable and less valuable, higher and lower life. (...) The most immediate fact in human consciousness is: 'I am life that wants to live, in the midst of life that wants to live'" (Schweitzer, 2003, p. 398).

The contemporary theologian and church critic Eugen Drewermann, who deals with modern political and moral issues and also comments on animal ethics, follows this tradition and assumes an inseparable connection between the fate of man and animal.

Regardless of compassion and theological considerations, the contemporary American philosopher and most famous representative of deontological animal ethics, Tom Regan, extends Kant's principle to animals. Regan defines mammals, birds, and possibly fish, just like humans, as *subjects-of-a-life* and, hence, as part of the moral community:

"In my understanding, the moral community consists of exactly those beings that are of direct moral significance—those that [...] are to be morally considered" (Regan in Blesch et al., 2007, p. 72).

A subject-of-a-life is capable of having desires and of pursuing them with corresponding actions. It has memories, an emotional life, preferences, it has a psychological-physical identity and experiences well-being or discomfort. According to Regan, all subjects-of-a-life have the same *inherent value*, regardless of whether they belong to the human or another animal species. The inherent value of a being inevitably leads to this being having certain *rights*:

"If I treat you [the reader] as if you belong to the same category as an umbrella or a banana—that is, as if you are a thing that has no value beyond my [...] desires or purposes, I treat you wrongly. I treat you as if you were a something, when in truth you are a someone" (ibid., p. 78).

Rights are understood here as a claim to considerate treatment and also as a right not to be instrumentalized for the purposes of others. Thus, Regan's animal ethics implies the principled rejection of animal use practices.

2.2.3   Synergistic Approach

A third animal ethics approach is the *synergistic approach* of the American philosopher Peter Wenz. This attempts to unite the human interests of anthropocentrism and the moral insights of non-anthropocentrism. It is a pragmatic approach that tries to place animal rights within the reality of today's industrial conditions.

Wenz argues that considering the well-being of animals does not necessarily mean a decrease in human well-being, but on the contrary, it can even increase it—if the social context is taken into account. For example, he advocates for the abolition of factory farming, as it also harms humans, but for the continuation of killing animals in the context of so-called pest control.

Wenz summarizes the relationship between human and non-human interests as follows:

> "Just as people are happier when they stop thinking about their own happiness and do something for the sake of the matter, people flourish when they stop trying to extract the greatest possible benefit from nature and instead adopt a respectful attitude towards the non-human—an attitude that encourages a life that knows its limits." (Wenz in Blesch et al., 2007, p. 146)

Wenz's approach is an attempt to connect two seemingly contrary interests—namely the immediate interest in prosperity, well-being, and satisfaction of needs, and the moral interest in correct behavior towards non-human animals. In this search for a compatibility of two supposedly contrary interests, this approach represents a step in the right direction. In order to improve the living reality of animals, not just in thought and writing in utopias, but instead, it is necessary to transfer the insights of animal ethics into everyday life, into laws, and into everyday human behavior. And Wenz provides a coherent basis for discussion.

This brief introduction to some currents in the field of animal ethics is to be understood as a first overview of the complex topic. I therefore recommend to every practitioner in the field of animal-assisted therapy both a deeper reading of the standard works on animal ethics (for example, Singer, 1996) and an openness to new insights from the field of philosophy and related sciences for discourse on moral values in dealing with animals (for example, Joy, 2013). In the following section, based on the insights of animal ethics, I formulate questions for the discipline of animal-assisted therapy, which the field in general and every practitioner in particular should deal with.

2.3   What Specific Questions Does Animal Ethics Raise for Animal-Assisted Therapy?

There are numerous questions that animal ethics raises for practical and everyday coexistence with animals. With regard to animal-assisted therapy, as it typically looks today, it ultimately comes down to the central question of whether humans may use animals as a means to achieve a defined purpose. More precisely, the question is:

- If we assume that animal-assisted therapy aims to increase human well-being through the use of animals, and that the animals must accept certain restrictions of their natural expressions and limitations of their individual needs for this—*may we then use animals in human therapy*?

Let's consider this question in light of the different representatives of animal ethics that I introduced in the previous chapter. If we, like Regan, assume that animals are subjects-of-a-life, i.e., individuals with desires, needs, fine perception, and personalities, then it is not ethically correct to use them as a means to an end. Regan formulates it as follows:

> "Sentient beings are not treated with respect (their rights are violated) when they are treated as mere means to promote the interests or fulfill the desires of others." (Regan in Blesch et al., 2007, p. 87).

If we refer to Singer, the answer is also negative: Based on the principle of equality, the interests of human and non-human animals have the same significance, so it is not ethically correct to subordinate the interests of animals to the interests of humans.

Although Wenz always has human well-being in mind alongside the rights of animals, the answer is still negative. According to Wenz, humans can only truly benefit from contact with animals if they turn to them for their own sake:

> "The true path to happiness is to appreciate the activity, person, thing, or endeavor for its own sake, for its own significance. (…) For people to be well, they must care for animals for the sake of the animals, without constantly referring to human well-being." (Wenz in Blesch et al., 2007, p. 141).

In summary, it can be stated: From the perspective of animal ethics, it is wrong to use animals in the therapy of humans under the stated premises (i.e., increasing human well-being associated with a restriction of animals).

Does this mean that the use of animals in the therapy of humans must generally be avoided? No, it does not. The problem from an animal ethics perspective is not the fact that the animals help humans, but the objective and conditions under which this happens.

▶   **Important!** Animal-assisted therapy is to be criticized from an animal ethics perspective if animals are used as a means to an end without the animals themselves benefiting from their deployment. The problem is thus not the fact that the animals help humans, but the usual objective and the conditions for the animals.

If we change the objective and conditions in such a way that not only human interests count, but the interests of the animals are *equally valuable*, then the question and consequently the answer change:

- If we assume that animal-assisted therapy aims to increase both human well-being *and the well-being of the animals* and *the animals are allowed to maintain their natural expressions and their individual needs are respected*—may we then use animals in human therapy?

Based on Singer's utilitarian approach, we can clearly answer with *Yes*. If an action increases the well-being of all parties involved, then all sides benefit in a classic win-win situation, and the action is to be judged as ethically correct.

With Regan, the answer under these new conditions is also *Yes*. Because the animals are no longer a means to an end, but are perceived as subjects with needs and interests that carry the same weight as human interests and needs.

And Wenz's synergistic approach also answers the question with *Yes*, because exactly what Wenz postulates occurs: the interests of humans and the interests of animals are linked, and the long-term and actual well-being of humans is only increased when the well-being of animals is also increased.

So, when we humans use animals in therapy, we have the duty to make this use ethically correct towards the animal. Both *in* the therapy session, as well as *before and after each therapy session* and also *before we even start the therapy*—namely already in the selection of the animals and in their training. In the following section, I will now explain how it is possible to meet the ethical conditions for the use of animals in the context of animal-assisted therapy and thus offer good therapy for all involved.

Summary: Are we allowed to use animals in human therapy from an ethical point of view?

From an animal ethics perspective, humans are allowed to use animals in therapy, but this use is subject to certain conditions and obligations. Namely:

- The animals themselves must benefit from the animal-assisted therapy
- The animals must be allowed to retain their natural forms of expression
- The animals must be allowed to live out their individual needs

References

Animal Equality Germany e. V. (2019). www.animalequality.de. Accessed: 12. July 2019.
Blesch, K., Breunig, A., Buss, S., Dondaines, G., Ebert, R., Fruth, F., Kessler, N., Müller, M., Panten, U., Reimelt, A., Schälling, B., Schneele, J., Sixt-Sailer, A., Unger, M., & Zehmisch, A. (Eds.). (2007). *Tierrechte—Eine interdisziplinäre Herausforderung*. Harald Fischer.
Hatkoff, A. (2009). *The inner world of farm animals—Their amazing social, emotional, and intellectual capacities*. Stewart, Tabori & Chang.
Joy, M. (2013). *Warum wir Hunde lieben, Schweine essen und Kühe anziehen. Karnismus—Eine Einführung*. Compassion Media.
Kundera, M. (1988). *Die unerträgliche Leichtigkeit des Seins*. Fischer Taschenbuch.
Schweitzer, A. (2003). In C. von Günzler, U. Luz & J. Zürcher (Eds.), *Vorträge, Vorlesungen, Aufsätze—Werke aus dem Nachlass*. Beck.
Singer, P. (1996). *Animal Liberation—Die Befreiung der Tiere*. Rowohlt Taschenbuch.
Statista. (2019). https://de-statista.com/themen/174/haustiere. Accessed: 23. Sept. 2019.

My Concept of Good Animal-Assisted Therapy

3

Contents

Abstract

When we decide to apply animal-assisted therapy, we are faced with ethical obligations towards our animal. We have not only to preserve its right of well-being, but also bear the responsibility to ensure that the animal can benefit from the therapy. To achieve this, we have to consider various aspects, and this chapter is about these. First, it is clarified that the course of a good therapy from the animal's point of view is

K. Blesch, *Animal-Assisted Therapy with Dogs*,
https://doi.org/10.1007/978-3-662-67965-4_3

set long before we actually start working with the animal. In addition, animal-friendly implementation is not limited to the daily therapy use, but extends far beyond into all areas of life and all phases of the animal's life. The following therefore describes all relevant areas and their specific design that encompass the ethically correct implementation of good animal-assisted therapy.

It should be mentioned at this point that in the following explanations I will no longer speak of animals in general, but of dogs, as I mainly work with dogs, and this book is about working with dogs. However, I would like to emphasize that the discussed aspects of selection and training fundamentally also apply to all other types of animals used in therapy. Every animal—whether dog, rabbit or goat—has a right to a therapy that is *good* from its point of view.

3.1   Animal Welfare Comes First

Before we proceed to the selection, training, and specific deployment, let's establish the most important maxim of good animal-assisted therapy: As an animal-assisted therapist, you are always primarily responsible for the unconditional well-being of your animal, and only in the second, subsequent step, for the enhancement of the participant's well-being.

This arises from the discussions on animal ethics and the derived insight that the animal must also benefit from the animal-assisted therapy. Since the animal cannot speak for itself and thus cannot demand and ensure its own well-being, the therapist must reliably and consistently take over this role. If the therapist does not maintain the well-being of the animal, does not ensure that the animal is completely well, then no one does. The animal is completely dependent, and this fact must be acknowledged by setting animal welfare as the highest priority.

This attitude should be the supporting and unshakeable foundation of one's own work. The well-being of the animal always comes first. Once this is secured, the animal can be used to enhance the well-being of a patient or participant through therapy. This fact is the beginning of every animal-assisted work and must be constantly reinforced as an attitude. As will become apparent in the course of this chapter, this attitude can be challenged by various situations, such as external expectations (see Sect. 3.5) or the necessary retirement of the animal (see Sect. 3.9). Therefore, it is all the more important to constantly remind oneself of this clear priority and to consciously maintain it.

▶   **Important!** As an animal-assisted therapist, you are always primarily responsible for the unconditional well-being of your animal, and only in the second subsequent step for the enhancement of the participant's well-being.

3.2 Selection of the Dog

Everyone follows different principles when selecting a dog. Sometimes a dog comes to its human by chance, for example, because a friend's family dog has puppies or through an advertisement in the newspaper. In the following, I will present the aspects that are personally important to me when I am looking for a new dog. Specifically, I follow these three basic principles when selecting my dogs:

- Mixed breed dog instead of purebred dog
- Adopting instead of buying
- Pack instead of single dog

I will explain the reasons for this in the following sections.

3.2.1 Mixed Breed Dog Instead of Purebred Dog

Personally, I particularly appreciate mixed breed dogs. I enjoy it when chance determines the appearance and character of a dog, and the dog is not created through human grids, planning, and interventions.

Beyond this personal preference, there are also general aspects to consider when it comes to the difference between mixed breed and purebred dogs. Perhaps the following arguments will serve to question the prevailing opinion that purebred dogs are superior to mixed breed dogs, and instead to recognize the uniqueness of mixed breed dogs. The final decision on which dog to choose is up to each individual.

3.2.1.1 No Substantial Behavioral Differences Between Different Dog Breeds

It is often implicitly or explicitly assumed that the behavior of different dog breeds differs and that there are therefore breeds that are particularly suitable for therapy. Golden Retrievers, for example, are considered particularly loving family dogs and thus suitable therapy companion dogs. Terriers are considered particularly active and lively, Spitz dogs are suspicious of strangers—just to name a few common ideas.

These opinions are reinforced by statements suggesting that certain dog breeds are allegedly more intelligent than all others. For instance, Coren (1997) asked several hundred judges of dog obedience competitions about their personal assessment of the intelligence of different breeds and published a list of the most intelligent and least intelligent dog breeds based on this. According to this ranking, the Border Collie, the Poodle, and the Golden Retriever are among the most intelligent dog breeds. On the other hand, the Mastiff, the Beagle, and the Afghan are considered less intelligent. Anyone familiar with intelligence research or research in general will immediately recognize that some aspects of this survey do not meet the standards. Without going into all the details, the fundamental mistake is equating intelligence with obedience. A dog obeys and quickly learns new commands—hence, it is intelligent. If we were to apply this to humans, it would mean: someone who always immediately understands what is expected of them and carries it out promptly is intelligent; whereas someone who asks questions first or is more stubborn is stupid. I don't know anyone who would accept this definition of intelligence. Because: Intelligence is much more than understanding and implementing commands! In relation to dogs, we can assume at least three aspects of intelligence: on the one hand, *obedience intelligence*, i.e., how well a dog understands human instructions and follows them. But on the other hand, and beyond that, also the *instinctive intelligence,* which includes the purpose for which a dog was bred (so every type of dog will be better at things that correspond to its original area of use) and the *adaptive intelligence*, i.e., a dog's adaptability to its living conditions. Although it is now clear that Coren's survey was solely about the obedience of dogs and not their intelligence, it continues to haunt the popular science media world.

Serious research on the differences between various dog breeds, on the other hand, reveals different results. A meta-analysis of existing studies on this topic shows that so far, *no substantial, no consistent, and no predictable differences* in the behavior of different breeds have been found (Mehrkam & Wynne, 2014). This may sound surprising, as each of us has ideas about the behavior of certain dog breeds in mind. And the actual purpose of breeds is indeed to create predictable differences. But beware: Breeding was often and still is primarily based on appearance, and in most cases, the character of the dog is only considered secondarily (exceptions prove the rule)!

This leads to the fact that only minor reliable differences can be found regarding the behavior of different dog breeds. In terms of important characteristics such as willingness and ability to learn, openness towards strangers, friendliness, no significant differences between different dog breeds can be identified in studies. The reason for this is that the differences between individual dogs of the same breed are too large to attribute certain behaviors to a specific breed. Specifically, this means: There are Golden Retrievers who approach strangers openly and joyfully, are playful and tolerant, and are therefore well suited as therapy companion dogs, but there are also other Golden Retrievers who do not have these characteristics and would therefore not be suitable therapy companion dogs. The same applies to other breeds. Individual breeding associations and individual convinced breeders naturally claim otherwise, but the sober state of research clearly shows that the mere belonging to a certain dog breed is not a reliable predictor and certainly not a guarantee for certain character traits of a dog. Instead, studies suggest that differences between dogs, for example in terms of their problem-solving skills, are mainly due to practice and training (Marshall-Pescini et al., 2016). In summary, we can assume that behavioral differences in dogs are more influenced by learning experiences and training than by their breed affiliation.

▶   **Important!** The mere belonging of a dog to a certain breed indeed determines its appearance, but it is **no guarantee** for certain desired behaviors or character traits! Studies rather show that differences between individual dogs in terms of, for example, their problem-solving skills are primarily determined by their learning experiences and training, not by their breed affiliation.

3.2.1.2 Genetic Variability of Mixed Breed Dogs

Mixed breed dogs are less susceptible to recessively inherited diseases anchored in a dog's genetics than purebred dogs (Breeding Business, 2018). Of course, there are exceptions and mixed breed dogs also suffer from hereditary diseases. Sometimes it is argued that the disadvantage with mixed breed dogs is that there is no controlled intervention through breeding, and therefore hereditary diseases cannot be strategically eliminated. To understand the topic precisely, a look at Mendel's laws of inheritance helps.

Humans create a certain dog breed through breeding by reducing the variability of the gene pool of these dogs through artificial selection. In doing so, they strive for the desired similarity of the members of this breed in terms of certain characteristics. At the same time, this restriction of the gene pool automatically means that recessively inherited diseases become more likely. An English study found that ten out of twenty-four genetically inherited diseases are more likely in purebred dogs than in mixed breed dogs (Breeding Business, 2018). A 2014 study shows an increased likelihood for three out of twenty hereditary diseases in purebred dogs (O'Neill et al., 2014).

Other studies show no significant differences in terms of vet visits or life expectancy between mixed breed and purebred dogs (Switzer & Nolte, 2007). However, further studies are needed that include additional factors. For example, aspects such as: Does the mixed breed dog come from a shelter? Has it previously lived on the street? I hypothesize that factors such as previous poor nutrition, untreated diseases, and the like affect the otherwise robust health of a mixed breed dog and thus reduce the advantage that mixed breeds have due to their genetic variability in terms of health and life expectancy. However, this is speculation at this point and would need to be investigated in further studies.

Furthermore, it would be necessary to distinguish more precisely among the mixed breed dogs participating in a comparative study whether it is a mixed breed that was also created by direct or indirect human intervention in the dogs' reproduction, for example, a Labrador-German Shepherd mix, whose mother was a Labrador Retriever and whose father was a German Shepherd. Or whether it is a dog whose ancestors were not purebred dogs.

3.2.1.3 Underestimated Street Dogs

The dogs, whose ancestors were not purebred, are very interesting characters who, in my opinion, have so far been given far too little space in research. They have the most diverse names: "Pemba" dogs, village dogs, descendants of the original dogs, etc. What is meant are the so-called street dogs, the strays. The dogs, who are still often unjustly regarded as inferior.

The biologist Ray Coppinger has taken a closer look at these dogs and advocates for a rethink in our understanding of breed and origin of dogs:

> "Mongrels are usually considered a kind of degenerate dog, which is a crossbreed of different breeds. The general view is that these dogs all descend from purebred ancestors. When we see a mixed breed, we immediately try to find out which breeds have been incorporated into it. It took me years to realize that a dog does not necessarily have to be a crossbreed of breeds if it does not look like a purebred dog" (Coppinger & Coppinger, 2013, p. 71).

Coppinger has observed populations of street dogs, among others in Tanzania, and concludes that these dogs are to be classified as direct descendants of the original dogs. He further assumes that "similar populations of early village dogs were the beginning of the development of modern breeds" (ibid., p. 87).

Instead of assuming inferiority compared to a purebred dog, it would instead be appropriate to learn to appreciate the uniqueness of these dogs. I myself have had experiences with these dogs and have the utmost respect for their origin, their survivability, and their nature, which is often characterized by a high level of serenity and ability to be autonomous. A certain similarity in nature is due to the living conditions to which they are exposed through their own life and the life of their ancestors (ibid.). These dogs live indirectly with humans, are part of human society and at the same time they are responsible for their own survival. This results in them being able to assess humans and human moods well, as this is vital for a street dog. In addition, they are independent and autonomous dogs. Cleo, as a former street dog, for example, continued to pull earthworms out of the ground and eat them on walks in the first weeks after her adoption. To this day, Cleo sets up a sleeping place in the undergrowth or bushes whenever we linger a little longer at one place on a walk. She pushes aside sticks, digs a small hollow and always chooses a well-camouflaged spot for her place. These are just two examples that show how well former street dogs as Cleo can provide for their own food and find and set up a safe sleeping place. These dogs can also calm themselves down very well, are independent and yet very pack-minded and loyal. These are all abilities that I highly value in a dog and that, in my experience, make living together with these dogs colorful and instructive.

3.2.2   Adopt Don't Shop

Animal welfare organizations highlight the paradoxical situation of dogs in today's world by pointing out the contradiction between increasingly full animal shelters and rising breeding numbers. Every year, more and more dogs are surrendered to animal shelters, while at the same time more and more dogs are brought onto the market (Peta, 2013). Thanks to various exposé reports, it is now probably undisputed that buying puppies from pet stores or over the internet is not recommended. As a buyer, the living conditions of the animals cannot be checked, so it is uncertain whether the puppies are health-compromised or "overbred"[1] . There is also the risk of supporting criminally operating organizations or at least unscrupulous individuals with the purchase of the puppies, who are only interested in profitable distribution of the puppies at the expense of the health and well-being of the animals.

However, even reputable breeders and recognized breeding associations are at least critically viewed from an animal ethics perspective. Although the dogs usually grow up healthy and in species-appropriate conditions, everyone should be aware that the active breeding of dogs reduces the chances of rehoming surrendered dogs: "Even those who buy a dog or a cat from a "small" breeder are not acting in the interest of animal welfare. Every animal from the shelter is denied a real chance of a new home through this purchase. […] anyone who absolutely wants a young animal or an animal of a certain "breed" will find what they are looking for in the animal shelter or on private foster care sites and therefore does not have to promote the "production" of animals, while countless animals are already waiting for a home." (Peta, 2013)

Since there are still some prejudices and fears regarding the adoption of a dog from animal welfare—especially when someone wants to work with the dog—I will dedicate a separate chapter to this topic later in the book. Here I will explain what to specifically look for when choosing a dog from animal welfare.

3.2.3 Pack Instead of Lone Dog

Most dogs benefit from living with a fellow canine. The prerequisite is that the two or more dogs like each other, and that none of the dogs feel neglected. If these conditions are met, most dogs benefit from living with one or more fellow canines. This gives them the opportunity to occasionally disconnect from the human world, to communicate naturally, or to play wildly. Because even if we humans strive for successful communication with the dog, allow him his dog language and respond to him and his needs, we still cannot completely replace a "canine" communication partner or playmate (see Fig. 3.1).

And from a professional point of view, I can only strongly advise anyone who wants to work in the field of animal-assisted therapy to have at least two therapy companion dogs. This is the only way to conserve the dogs' working power and to deal flexibly and relaxedly with issues such as breaks or retirement of one of the dogs. If one of the dogs retires—and retirement means that the dog no longer works, but of course continues to live happily in his family—the other dog is still ready for action, and you can calmly prepare a third dog for his deployment in parallel (see Fig. 3.2). This is only briefly mentioned here, more on this in the further course of the chapter (Sect. 3.9).

---

[1] Overbreeding is a vague term. In this context, it means that a lot of offspring are produced in the course of breeding, with too little attention paid to genetic diversity, resulting in a significantly increased risk of hereditary diseases in the offspring.

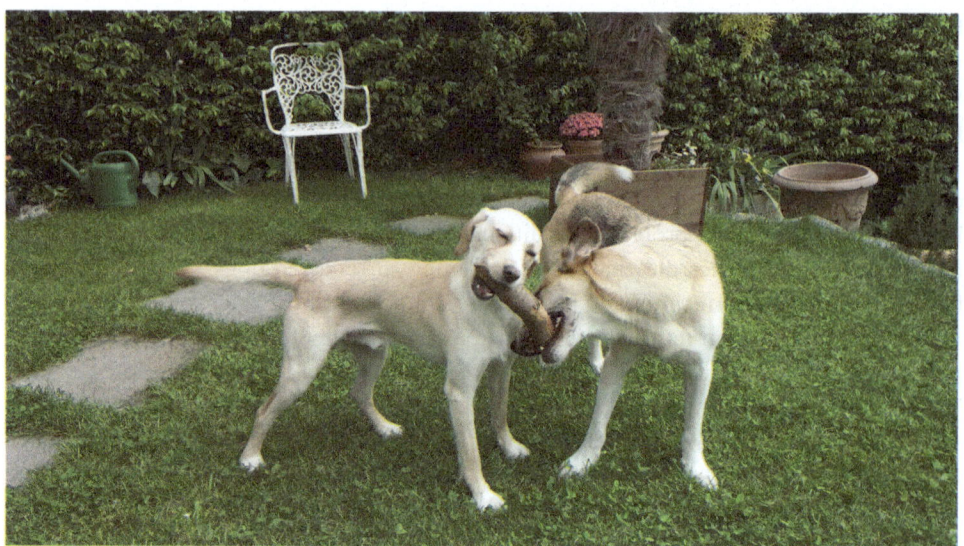

Fig. 3.1 Play among dogs

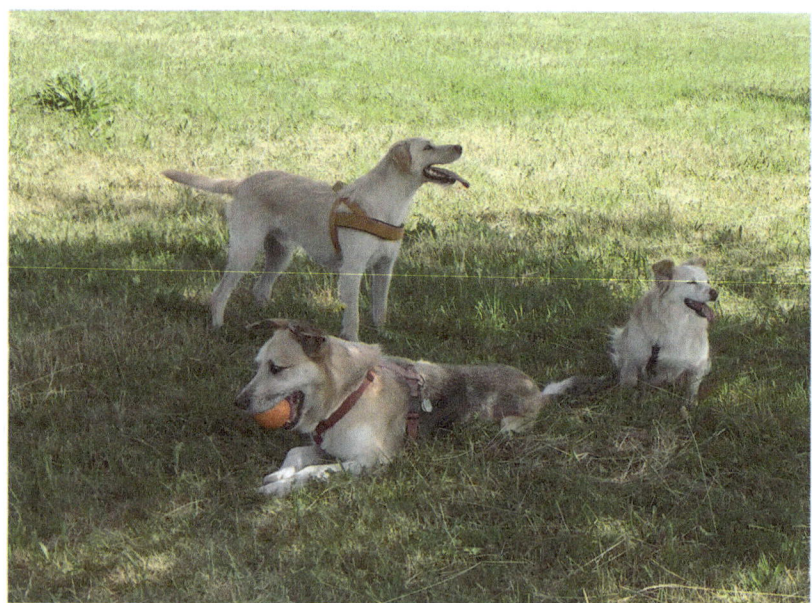

Fig. 3.2 Cleo, Giulio and Toni after training

When keeping several dogs, it is important to maintain a certain hierarchy among the dogs. Personally, I handle it in such a way that the hierarchy is determined by the time of admission into the family. Currently, this means: first Giulio, then Cleo, then Toni. This applies, for example, when feeding, rewarding, or leashing. The hierarchy among the dogs can also be established differently, but I find the regulation according to arrival most sensible, because it gives the dogs, who suddenly have to share their resources with the newcomer, the security of not losing anything to "the new one". This security is necessary for the dogs to interact peacefully with each other. In all the years with several dogs and sometimes very different characters, there were never any significant conflicts between my dogs due to this clear structure. They know when it's their turn and can therefore relax and live peacefully together.

3.3 Choosing the Right Training

The step following the selection of the dog is the decision about the type and manner of the dog's upbringing or training. So far, there are no universally valid, binding rules for the implementation of animal-assisted therapy, because the term and the activity are unfortunately not yet protected. Currently, there are only various certificates from different institutes, and anyone who wants to have their work certified by one of these institutes must adhere to the corresponding guidelines and examination regulations. Anyone who now wants to further educate themselves or their dog in parallel to a seminar or training course is faced with a veritable flood of literature on correct dog training. In addition, there are numerous dog schools and dog trainers who offer seminars, courses, mobile training hours.

This immense growth in the field of dog training in recent years can certainly be seen as positive, as every dog owner now has the opportunity to inform themselves, further their education, and learn. At the same time, the sheer number of guides and the competition between different dog trainers quickly lead to uncertainty among dog owners. What is described as correct in one guide is presented as a mistake in dog training in the next guide. What one dog trainer recommends, the next dog trainer categorically rejects. Examples of such contradictions can be found in all areas of living together with a dog and thus range from rewarding (never with treats versus always with treats) and command giving (sharp command versus only visual signals) to the dog's sleeping habits (dog must sleep in a transport box versus dog can sleep wherever it wants). What already makes private dog owners uncertain, often greatly irritates prospective practitioners in the field of animal-assisted therapy.

Which dog school, which training path should one choose if one wants to prepare one's dog appropriately for use in animal-assisted therapy?

In addition to basic aspects such as the seriousness of those responsible and the use of exclusively non-violent training methods, in my experience, the most important criteria for choosing a training path are that the dog has *fun during training*, and that the training *promotes the dog in its individuality*. In terms of the dog's enjoyment of training, this means specifically: The dog should go to the training area with joy, have fun with the exercises, and leave the area satisfied at the end of training. Regarding the promotion of individuality, this means that the training should aim to recognize and respond to the individual character of the dog. Too often, there is an attempt to impose a certain training method on every dog—regardless of the dog's individual temperament and nature.

It is important to recognize what the dog likes to do, what it is good at, and what it is passionate about. These aspects should be promoted in good training. A lively, active dog can easily be excited for games of any kind and can learn, for example, to reliably return through this. A "greedy" dog is best rewarded with treats and can learn the command "down" well with this help, for example.

Of course, the dog should also learn to do certain things that it does not (yet) like to do on its own. An active dog, for example, must learn to be able to relax and lie down quietly. It should learn this not least for its own sake, as it is particularly beneficial for very active dogs to learn to relax. This learning of new behaviors or behaviors that are not yet part of the dog's spontaneous behavior repertoire should happen slowly and at an appropriate pace for the dog. It is important not to frustrate or overwhelm the dog in this process.

And again: The main focus of good training is always on what the dog offers on its own or what it is particularly enthusiastic about. It is not sensible to want to make a lively dog into a therapy companion dog that quietly lies down in a circle of chairs in a nursing home. This is constant work against the nature of this dog and is not appropriate to its needs. Similarly, it is not right to force a quiet, introverted dog into excessive activity.

Example: The training should promote the individuality of the dog

The three dogs I work with are very different. I recognize this difference in their training as well as in their daily work, so that each of them is rewarded differently and specializes in different tasks and exercises.

Giulio (Shepherd mix) loves treats above all. He interacts very finely with humans, pays attention to details, and is very attentive.

Reward for Giulio: treats; Exercises: interaction exercises

Cleo (Spitz mix) is cuddly and reacts enthusiastically to high pitches when spoken to. She moves concentrated and thoughtful, choosing her paths very carefully.

Reward for Cleo: vocal praise; Exercises: parcours work

Toni (Hunting dog mix) loves ball games. He loves to run passionately and searches with enthusiasm.

Reward for Toni: his ball; Exercises: movement and search games ◀

Checklist: What to consider when choosing the right dog school (the right dog trainer, the right training institute)?

- Seriousness
  - Provider has certified titles/diplomas as a dog trainer or similar
  - Provider has the required permission according to § 11 of the Animal Welfare Act (= the requested permission of the country you live in)
- Recommendation
  - Provider was recommended
  - or has a good overall reputation
- Gentle training methods
  - Provider uses exclusively non-violent training methods (no choke collar or similar)
- Transparent description of contents and methods
  - Provider openly describes his approach and his training methods
- You work with your dog in training
  - Provider instructs the dog owner; the owner performs the exercises with the dog himself
- The dog enjoys the training
  - He enjoys going to the training ground
  - He participates with joy
  - He is satisfied after the training
- The dog's individuality is recognized and the training is tailored to his individual nature
  - Reward is selected according to his preferences
  - Focus is on promoting what he offers on his own and/or what he is enthusiastic about
  - New behaviors (which may not correspond to his temperament) are built up slowly, without overwhelming the dog

3.4   Designing the Therapy so that the Dog also Enjoys It

If it were up to most dogs, they would choose to frolic in a meadow with their buddies or their humans, sniff the world, and then doze off comfortably curled up at home after a fine meal. Instead, fetching balls for various people in a nursing home or school, tolerating sharp and unpleasant smells like disinfectants and cleaning agents for the dog's nose, and at the same time being confronted with often strong human emotions, is significantly less attractive from a dog's perspective. Considering this and the claim that the dog should also enjoy the therapy (Sect. 2.3), it is therefore necessary to prepare and implement the therapy in such a way that the dog can live a long, healthy, and happy life and specifically enjoy the singular therapy sessions.

3.4.1   Creating a Dog-Friendly Environment

First and foremost, it is essential to create an environment in which the dog has access to everything it needs (water, rest opportunities), and it can feel as comfortable as possible. This is significantly easier in one's own premises than in visiting services or mobile work in foreign premises. Nevertheless, it is also possible here to make the environment as dog-friendly as possible by reducing potential unpleasant environmental factors. Ventilating before the session starts is very important. This reduces the aversive smells of disinfectants and cleaning agents or simply the "stale" and perhaps too warm room air in winter for the dog's nose. Most rooms where mobile animal-assisted therapy takes place have no carpet floors for hygiene reasons. In large or empty rooms, this can lead to an unpleasant echo. This can be reduced by bringing as many blankets and resting places as possible and laying them out in the room where possible. This dampens the echo for the sensitive dog's hearing and simultaneously creates a more familiar environment. Some of the provided accomodations, but at least one of them, should provide a retreat for the dog. It should therefore be positioned at a certain distance from the therapy field (the circle of chairs or the individual patient), perhaps under a table or in a corner. The dog can retreat here at any time and find some peace if it should need it.

When working in one's own premises, it is important to create real security for the dog. Here too, he should be offered at least one retreat and several resting places (see Fig. 3.3). In addition, it should be allowed that the room smells pleasant or at least neutral to the dog. This also means regular ventilation (for example, before and after each therapy session). It is also recommended not to wash the dog's blankets and beds too often. Of course, they should not smell unpleasant to the human nose, but it creates familiarity and security for the dog if they are allowed to carry his smell and are only washed when it is really necessary. It is therefore also necessary to clean the room with as neutral cleaning agents as possible.

3.4.2   Establish Clear Behavioral Rules Towards the Dog

After we have created a comfortable space, the therapy begins. For the therapy to start well for the dog, it is important to design the greeting of the participant(s) in a way that suits the nature of the dog. Some dogs greet happily and joyfully; other dogs are more reserved. Both are fine. Especially in the latter case, the dog should not be forced to do anything. If participants are disappointed about this, it is necessary to explain and make the behavior of the dog understandable to the participant. Moreover, participants often appreciate it when a initially reserved dog opens up and comes to them during the course of therapy (see Fig. 3.4).

During the therapy session, a pleasant noise level should be maintained, especially in group sessions. This is not always easy depending on the target group. But it can and should be part of the therapy for participants to learn to adapt their own behavior to the situation and not to violate the needs of others (in this case the needs of the dog). In my

Fig. 3.3 Giulio on one of his beds in the individual therapy setting

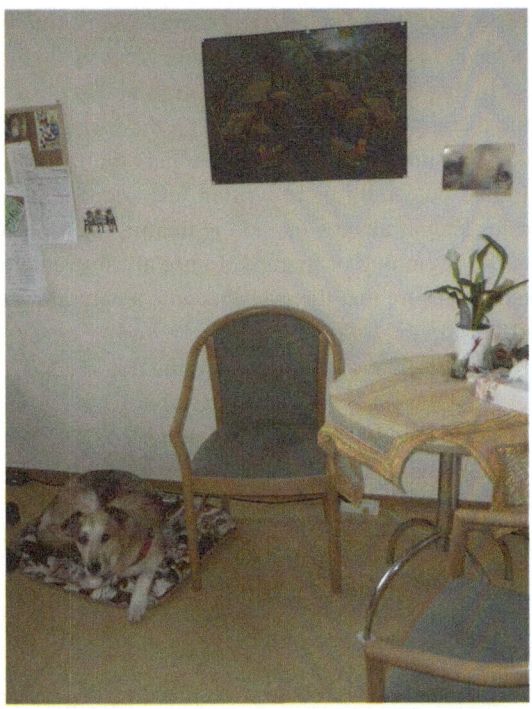

Fig. 3.4 Here two are fond of each other—accordingly intimate greeting

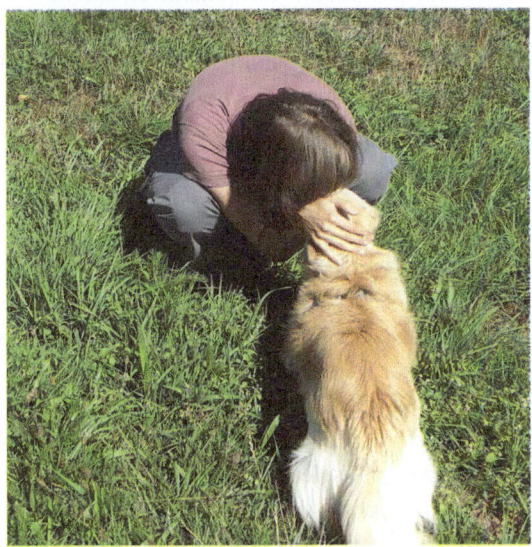

experience, even people with severe dementia are sometimes still able to regulate their behavior as to not frighten the dog (Blesch, 2013).

In this context, it is helpful to establish clear behavioral rules towards the dog before the therapy begins. Depending on the participant, the dog, and the setting, these rules are of corse different. The example lists the rules that apply to my therapy setting and that I hand out orally or in written form depending on the participant. What the behavioral rules should always include is treating the dog with respect. Since rules discussed once at the beginning of therapy do not always remain present for the participant, it is important to ensure that the rules become a natural part of interaction. This can be achieved by observing the following:

The behavioral rules towards the dog are…

- made tangible and **understandable**,
- **justified** and their importance is made clear,
- regularly **repeated**,
- asserted firmly and kindly **enforced** if they are not observed.

Example: Behavioral rules towards dogs, as I comunicate them to the participants of the animal-assisted therapy

- **Respect for the dog**: We meet the dog at eye-to-eye level and respect its boundaries
- **Perception of the dog as an individual**: We perceive the dog as an individual with its own needs, its own character, and its own will, and treat it accordingly
- **Working with the dog is working on ourselves**: We use the exchange with the dog to learn something about ourselves. Through its behavior, the dog continuously gives us unadulterated feedback about how we affect it. In our relationship with the dog, we have the opportunity to reflect on ourselves and change our behavior. ◀

3.4.3 Dog-Friendly and Therapeutically Meaningful Exercises

In order for the dog to enjoy the therapy itself, activities should be chosen that the dog likes and that fit the respective context. In general, any activity can be designed and accompanied in such a way that the participant can enjoy it. This is the task of the therapist. Therefore, when selecting games or exercises with the dog, it should be the case that the therapist selects these in the interest of the dog and then makes them attractive for the participant.

In reality, however, it is sometimes the case that the therapist asks the participant what they would like to do today, and then the participant chooses something from a range of suggestions (throwing and fetching a ball, petting, searching for treats, having a specific toy fetched by the dog, and so on), and this game is then played with the dog. It is

assumed that the dog will somehow enjoy it. After all, he knows the game and participates. However, there are some *fallacies* in this.

The first fallacy or mistake is that the choice of exercise is left to the participant. Letting the participant decide what they would like to do is *not* therapy. Therapy means that
the therapist sets a specific goal with the participant, and then works towards it in a structured way. These can be the most varied goals, depending on the area in which animal-
assisted therapy is applied. In the context of psychotherapy, for example, it will be the
enhancement of self-esteem or self-confidence. In the context of occupational therapy,
for example, it could be general activation or the improvement of motor skills. In the
context of animal-assisted therapy, the exercises with the dog are not an end in themselves, but should be designed in such a way that the participant can practice a certain
behavior or action through them.

The therapist therefore selects the exercises. If, for example, the goal of the animal-
assisted therapy is to activate the participant, then the exercises should challenge the
participant mentally and physically within his or her capabilities. There can be a certain degree of freedom in this by allowing the participant to choose between two similar
exercises. However, if the participant is allowed to choose from a pool of possibilities,
then the participant will unconsciously or consciously stay in his or her *comfort zone*,
i.e., choose an exercise that he or she can already do, that is easy for him or her, and that
therefore demands little or nothing from him or her.

▶   **Important!** Therapy means that the therapist selects the content of the sessions
        and thus the exercises with the dog in the interest of the individual goal of the par-
        ticipant. Allowing the participant to freely decide what they would like to do with
        the dog is *not* therapy.

The second mistake is that the exercise is carried out by the dog and the participant and
the therapist is not present enough. I cannot repeat often enough that in animal-assisted
therapy, the therapist is the therapist and not the dog or the animal. This means: interaction takes place with the dog, and the task of the therapist is to turn this interaction
into therapy. Throwing a ball to a dog may be a nice activity, but it is not yet therapy.
This interaction becomes therapy when the therapist provides assistance and guidance
so that the participant can work on his or her general problem through this activity. If the
patient suffers from physical limitations, he or she is encouraged to throw "for the dog"
as far and powerfully as possible. In this way, the participant is motivated to engage in
physical activity and push their limits through the game with the dog. If a participant,
on the other hand, suffers from a lack of self-confidence, and the goal of the therapy is
to increase this, then the therapist will guide the exercise differently. Then it is not about
the performance of throwing far, but about the participant gradually gaining confidence
in their own actions. The therapist helps the participant to think constructively, reduce
fear of failure, and try something new in a playful way. The analysis before and after the
exercise with the dog is in the foreground; the technique and how far the ball is thrown

is completely irrelevant here. The therapist therefore needs to be continuously and intensively present. It must not happen that he or she steps back and lets the participant and the dog "just do it". This is a mere leisure activity for the participant and has nothing to do with therapy.

▶   **Important!** An exercise with the dog is never therapeutic per se.
An exercise with the dog becomes a therapeutic exercise *only if* the therapist…:

   … selects the exercise purposefully for the participant,
   … transparently explains why he chose the exercise and what relation this has to the participant's problem and therapeutic goal,
   … guides the exercise with suitable assistance for the participant,
   … discusses the exercise in relation to the individual problem of the participant,
   … and transfers what was learned in the exercise to other areas of the participant's life.

The third misconception is the assumption that the dog enjoys an activity in the therapy setting because he generally likes it. It may well be that the dog is cuddly and likes to be petted, but would prefer to keep more physical distance from a specific participant. This can have various reasons. For example, the individual smell of the participant may be unpleasant to the dog. Or the participant radiates tension and nervousness, which keeps the dog at distance. Therefore, it is important to have a good understanding of your own dog and to recognize how comfortable or uncomfortable he feels near the participant.

Does the dog spontaneously approach the participant or does he spontaneously keep his distance? Does he relax near the participant or does he become restless? Does the dog seek eye contact with me more often than usual while interacting with the participant?

If I know my dog well, I quickly get an impression of how comfortable or uncomfortable he feels in contact with a participant. At the same time, it is important to consider the dog's mood. If we ensure a healthy balance (see Sect. 3.7), we can assume that the dog is usually cheerful and calm. However, dogs also have bad days, have just experienced something exciting, or are tired. In order for the dog to also enjoy the therapy session, it is important to consider his relationship with the participant and his current condition, and to select the exercises based on this.

If the dog prefers to keep his distance from the participant, then interaction exercises without direct physical contact should be chosen, such as search games. The respective exercise is then adapted to the individual problem of the participant.

Example: Adapting a search exercise with the dog to the individual theme of the participant

An exercise is always the same only in its basic structure. The focus during the exercise, however, is always individual and oriented towards the theme of the participant and thus the therapeutic goal of the exercise. This is best illustrated by comparing the following two examples:

First, the general procedure of a search game:

The dog moves without a leash on the training ground. The participant calls the dog, who comes, then the participant throws a treat into a specific area of the ground and calls out "Search!". The dog finds the treat, is praised and called back. If the dog does not find the treat, it is helped by pointing out the correct area.

Varying focus of the search game illustrated by two examples:

Example 1

A participant is very performance-oriented in dealing with Toni. The goal of the therapy is to increase her general relationship competence, which specifically includes empathetic understanding of the dog and friendly interaction with him. The participant is encouraged to address Toni in a friendly voice, to call "Search!" as encouragingly as possible, and to follow Toni's search with her eyes. The focus is then primarily on praising Toni. Once he has found the treat, the challenge is to rejoice with him over his search success (empathetic understanding) and to praise him lovingly (kindness). This exercise challenges the participant's behavior patterns, as the instructions initially provoke some resistance from her. "Why should I praise the dog when he already gets a treat?" This sentence contains more implicit assumptions than one might initially think. It becomes clear that there is an internal aversion to praising the dog "too much", and at the same time there is a devaluation of the importance of one's own praise: The treat is more important and sufficient; one's own praise is relatively insignificant. The more self-confidence the participant develops in the course, the more generous she is with her praise, the more she enjoys the dog's success, and the more she expresses her connection to the dog through spontaneous, joyful exclamations during their shared play.

Example 2

A young man participates in animal-assisted self-confidence training. He suffers from low self-esteem, having experienced various setbacks in education and career. He is currently unemployed and has no professional perspective. The therapeutic goal is to activate and increase the feeling of self-efficacy. In the search game, I therefore focus on the participant learning to conduct the game in a concentrated, motivated, and healthy ambitious manner. It often happens during the search that Toni does not immediately find a treat. If clever Toni then notices that the participant is not really involved, that he doesn't care whether he finds it or not, then Toni only searches superficially, comes back on his own and "asks" for a new treat. So we practice "sticking to it", even if success does not come immediately. The motto in this case is to consistently motivate Toni to keep searching and not to give up, no matter how long it takes.

The same exercise has a completely different focus in the two presented cases. The focus is determined by the individual goal of the participant and is expressed in my instructions and in the analyses and discussions about the exercises. ◄

If the dog is a bit tired for some reason, I will reduce his involvement that day by, for example, reading a therapeutic story (preferably with a dog as the protagonist) that fits the participant's problem area, or incorporating the mindful observation of the dog as a relaxation exercise.

▶   **Important!** Just because a dog likes to play ball or is cuddly in his free time, it explicitly does *not* mean that he also likes playing ball or being petted with the respective participant and/or on the respective day.

In order for the dog to also enjoy the therapy session, it is important to consider his relationship with the participant as well as his current condition and to select the exercises based on this.

In general, it is important—both in terms of therapy and in terms of conserving the dog's resources—to encourage the participant to perform exercises and activities mindfully and consciously. The participant learns various central things through a slow and conscious approach. By mindfully carrying out the exercises with the dog, the participant can learn…:

- … to pay attention to themselves and their actions,
- … to train their body awareness,
- … to better assess their external impact,
- … to better interpret the reactions of the dog,
- … to reduce performance thinking
- … and to focus on the relationship with the dog.

The last two points are often relevant in today's times. Many participants who come to me are shaped and burdened in one way or another by exaggerated performance thinking. Developing a counterweight to this in the course of working with the dog and consciously focusing on relationship building and maintenance, rather than on one's own performance or the performance of others (the dog), is a pleasant and also progressive experience for many. At the same time, this focus noticeably relieves the dog and also leads from the participant's perspective to the dog's well-being having the same relevance as the participant's enjoyment of the therapy.

Example: Moving away from performance thinking towards relationship maintenance

A participant comes into animal-assisted therapy with low self-esteem. As is not uncommon in adults with psychological stress, she was confronted with high performance demands by her parents as a child. She was praised for good academic performance; otherwise, she experienced little affection from her parents. In combination with professional demands, this has led to a pronounced fear of performance over the years. She sets high standards for herself, makes her self-esteem dependent on this, and is afraid of not meeting her performance expectations.

The participant's performance orientation also came into play in her interaction with Giulio. She focused her interest on performing an exercise with the dog as well as possible, which specifically involved running a slalom with him. The relationship with the dog as well as her own well-being and the well-being of the dog during the slalom were outside her spontaneous focus. It was about performance for her, i.e., that all pylons were run through evenly, not about the fun of it or the relationship with Giulio. And if a slalom course did not go as she had hoped, she felt bad and devalued herself. The therapy served to help the participant learn to consciously focus on the *how*. Instead of the rigid, perfect running of the slalom course, she should learn to focus on how she can create well-being for herself and Giulio during the run. She should run the slalom with a pleasant feeling in her stomach and Giulio with a wagging tail and joyful facial expression. It was explicitly irrelevant whether she missed a pylon or led Giulio asymmetrically through the course. It was not about performance, it was about the relationship and the fun of the common task. The participant was challenged by this change of focus, but was able to render her own feelings and experiences towards herself and Giulio increasingly benevolent over time. The performance thinking presentend itself briefly from time to time during therapy, and this gave us the opportunity to discuss dealing with one's own demands and expectations and to look for other, new ways of dealing with tasks. ◀

Checklist: How can we ensure that *the dog* also enjoys the therapy?
- In unfamiliar surroundings: Reduction of possible unpleasant environmental factors
  - Bring everything the dog needs (water bowl, toys, and so on)
  - Ventilate
  - Bring various blankets and resting places, lay them out in the room (dampens the echo of noises, creates familiarity)
  - Create retreats
- In own premises: Establish a sense of security
  - Have or bring everything the dog needs (water bowl, toys, and so on)
  - Create retreats

- – Offer multiple resting places
- – Allow the room to smell pleasant for the dog
  Do not wash blankets and spots too often
  Clean with as neutral cleaning agents as possible
- Give the dog time for his form of greeting
- Ensure a pleasant soundscape
- Establish and enforce clear behavioral rules towards the dog
- Choose activities that the dog enjoys
- Make participants aware of the activities, thereby the therapy effect is higher *and* the dog's resources are conserved

3.5   Courage to Make Unpopular Decisions for the Sake of the Animals

People who are physically or mentally burdened often feel uncomfortable with themselves and their environment. Or in other words: they have a high level of suffering. This suffering can lead to the affected person withdrawing into themselves, focusing more on themselves and their condition. Therefore, when we work with people with a high level of suffering, we should be aware that their empathy skills may be limited.

What this can mean for animal-assisted therapy is shown by the extreme example of so-called dolphin therapy (see Sect. 1.3). Dolphins are highly sensitive and intelligent wild animals with an immense urge to move and complex social structures. It is undisputed that dolphins cannot be happy if they are kept in small pools and trained for therapy purposes (reports, 2019). Nevertheless, people book this therapy because their suffering due to a physical or mental illness is very high. Unscrupulous individuals have built a lucrative business model on this suffering and continue to advertise for it despite increasing protests against this so-called therapy. Affected individuals and relatives, such as parents of seriously ill children, may grasp at any straw and spend a lot of money to travel to Turkey, the USA, or other countries for this offer. The example of dolphin therapy shows: If the suffering of those affected is very high, then empathy for the animal counterpart can be reduced.

In relation to animal-assisted therapy with dogs, this means: It may be that the participant has little insight into the limits and needs of the dog and, for example, desires a behavior from the dog that would overwhelm it. Baring this in mind, we as therapists are encouraged to dare and be ready to make even unpopular decisions in favor of our therapy companion animals.

Example: Making an unpopular decision in favor of the therapy dog

An unpopular decision could be, for example, to end a therapy prematurely or to limit the number of times certain exercises are performed because the dog is tired. I often experience that participants would like to repeat a successful exercise over and over again because they enjoy the sense of achievement. And I also experience the opposite, namely, that an exercise does not succeed for the participant, and he would like to repeat it until it succeeds, despite the dog's fatigue. In the first case, it is therapeutically sensible to limit the execution so that the participant can learn to consciously enjoy a sense of achievement, instead of always chasing after new confirmations. And in the second case, it is therapeutically just as important to limit the number of exercises. Here, it is about accepting and acknowledging failure and, on the other hand, about *set-up-for-success* (i.e., enabling success): To draw a line, to look at what went wrong and to approach the difficult exercise again in the next session, fresh and well-prepared, which is much more promising than to continue increasingly tense and without reflexion. ◄

In order to be able to make possibly necessary unpopular decisions, it is good to sensitize the participant to the limits of the dogs in terms of concentration from the very beginning. At the same time, the therapist must be able to say *no*. Being able to say no to the participant means nothing other than being able to set necessary boundaries in the interest of the dog. In this sense, the skill and willingness to say no sometimes is an important area of competence for the therapist. Anyone who feels primarily responsible for their animals will not find it difficult to set boundaries in the interest of their animals.

In case of difficulties with saying no, it can be helpful to keep in mind that as an animal-assisted therapist, you are first and foremost responsible for the unconditional well-being of your animal and only in the second step, building on this, for the well-being of the participant (see Sect. 3.1). Considering this, it should not be difficult to formulate a friendly and justified no, if necessary.

▶   **Important!** In case of difficulties with saying no, it is helpful to keep in mind that as an animal-assisted therapist, you are first and foremost responsible for the unconditional well-being of your animal and only in the second step, building on this, for the well-being of the participant.

The courage to make unpopular decisions in the interest of the dog is occasionally also needed in dealing with the client. Often, the client of animal-assisted therapy is not the participant himself, but a family member or an institution such as a nursing home or a clinic. As a rule, it can be assumed that the client has the increase in the well-being of his resident or patient in focus and initially does not ask any questions regarding the well-being of the animals used. Thus, the client does not question on his own whether the desired duration of the assignment would overwhelm the dog.

In my experience, there is also little awareness of how demanding the deployment actually is and how important breaks (Sect. 3.6) and the balance before and after the therapies (Sect. 3.7) are for the dog. I have experienced that it is implicitly assumed that a therapy dog is always ready for action and that the therapy automatically brings him joy. How much work for the dog and therapist lays beyond an assignment is only realized by most clients when this is clearly named ans explained by the therapist.

Therefore, in my experience, it is fundamental to clearly establish the limits of readiness, breaks, and necessary preparation and follow-up for the dogs before the start of the assignment and to demand these. On such a basis, more understanding and interest in animal welfare can be expected from the client during the course. However, since there is no guarantee for this understanding, the following also applies here: As an animal-assisted therapist, one is always and primarily responsible for the unconditional well-being of one's animals. Therefore, one should not be afraid to set boundaries in the interest of the animals and, if necessary, to make unpopular decisions.

▶   **Important!** The animal-assisted therapist creates a central foundation for himself and his therapy dogs when he makes the limits of readiness, the necessity of breaks, and the preparation and follow-up of the dogs very clear to the client from the beginning on. In the course of this, one should never lack the courage to implement these important things and—if necessary—to demand them.

3.6   Breaks

During animal-assisted therapy, it is extremely important to maintain sufficient breaks for the dog. But what are sufficient breaks? First, it is necessary to clarify what is meant by breaks. For the area of animal-assisted therapy, I assume three different types of breaks, namely *spontaneous breaks*, *necessary breaks*, and *regulated breaks*.

Spontaneous breaks are the moments when the dog independently withdraws from the therapy process—for example, by lying down on one of his more distant resting places. These breaks must always be possible for the dog. The dog must be allowed to withdraw at any time. Anyone who prevents these spontaneous breaks endangers the general motivation of the dog for his participation in animal-assisted therapy and his psychological well-being. This should be explained just as transparently to the participants, then the corresponding understanding can be expected. If this understanding is not given, the courage to make unpopular decisions must not be lacking here either (Sect. 3.5).

Some dogs do not spontaneously take a break. They either have not learned that they are allowed to withdraw, or they have a high *will-to-please,* i.e., a strong desire to please their human. These dogs then stay in the situation, even if it is actually too much for them, they are put under stress by something, or they would simply need a moment of rest. In such cases, it is very important to observe necessary breaks.

Excursion: *will-to-please* in dogs

The *will-to-please* is a behavior in dogs that can be translated as a desire to please or a desire to do right. It is ultimately the basic desire of a dog to want to please the human. Almost every dog has a certain will-to-please. However, dogs differ in the degree of expression. Typical signs of a high will-to-please are, for example, the frequent search for eye contact with their human, a rather low desire for autonomy, and the pronounced desire for praise or confirmation. Dogs with a high will-to-please are often very motivated to learn and thus also teachable.

However, too strong an expression of the will-to-please can also have negative effects. Such a dog can stand out due to nervousness or be more susceptible to stress, as he is always looking for confirmation from the human and in this endeavor tries out changing behaviors and, so to speak, "offers" them to the human.

Since the will-to-please is usually associated with interest in humans and with friendly behavior towards humans, it often occurs in therapy dogs. Special attention should be paid to the observance of breaks in therapy dogs with a high will-to-please. In addition, these dogs often have to be actively taught to do nothing as a balance to therapy or to occupy themselves alone or with other dogs.

Necessary breaks are the breaks set by the therapist as soon as the dog shows, more frequently than usual, so-called *appeasement signals*. To quickly recognize signs of stress and thus signs of a necessary break, the therapist must be well acquainted with the appeasement signals used by his dog. Each dog has different preferences here. One dog uses very clear appeasement signals for humans, such as licking over the snout. Another dog is more subtle and uses finer signals such as looking to the side, which can be overlooked quite easily in group therapy. As a therapist, you must therefore know your dog's individual appeasement signals very well and also know when he uses them in order to be able to order a break when these signals appear or increase in frequency.

Excursion: Appeasement signals or Calming Signals (according to Turid Rugaas, 2001)

We understand appeasement signals as behaviors in dogs that serve two purposes:

1) On the one hand, the dog *calms* itself with this behavior
2) On the other hand, he wants to *appease* his counterpart with this behavior

Appeasement signals can be, for example:

- Looking away or avoiding eye contact
- Turning away
- Increased sniffing
- Very slow movements
- Licking over the snout or smacking

There are numerous appeasement signals, with most dogs preferring certain specific signals. Appeasement signals are shown in situations where dogs:

- are uncertain,
- experience or expect/fear a conflict,
- feel uncomfortable
- or feel stress

In addition to the spontaneous and necessary breaks, there must of course be *regulated breaks* for the dog. The duration and frequency of these breaks depend on the individual setting of the therapy as well as on the general constitution of the dog and his daily condition. I therefore do not want to formulate exact numbers and times as universally valid. Nevertheless, a few basic rules can be established:

- Young and older dogs generally need more frequent and longer breaks than a dog in its prime.
- After group therapy, a dog often needs a longer break than after individual contact.
- After each individual session, the dog needs a break before interacting with the next participant.
- The length of the break must allow the dog to "shake off" what it has experienced in therapy and to calm down.
- The quality of the break is more important than the duration.

What constitutes a high-quality break? In every therapy, the dog absorbs emotions and impressions. A good break should serve to allow the dog to process and "shake off" these emotions and impressions. So, if he has just had a session with a melancholic participant, exuberant frolicking might be a good break activity (see Fig. 3.5). On the other hand, if the dog has been working concentrated and actively, a relaxing petting session might be a sensible counterbalance to the experience. If the dog has had contact with various people, he might need rest and a nap the most (see Fig. 3.6). The content of the break should therefore be determined from the dog's perspective based on the previous experience and form a balancing counterweight to it.

▶ **Important!** The content of a good break should be determined from the dog's perspective based on the previous experience and form a balancing counterweight to it.

3.7   Before and After: Creating Balance

Outside of his role as a therapy companion, a therapy dog, like any human worker, also has a private life. This private life is lived with the dogs reference person, who should always be the person with whom the dog works. The dog should therefore live with the animal-assisted therapist. And our task as animal-assisted therapists is to enable the dog to live a happy life. What constitutes a happy life from a dog's perspective? The basis is that the dog feels like a loved part of the family, regardless of whether this family consists of the therapist and the dog or of several members. As a pack animal, every dog needs this feeling of belonging and security. For a therapy dog, who is confronted daily with changing people and strong emotions, this feeling of being cared for is particularly important as a balance.

Fig. 3.5 Active break in the forest

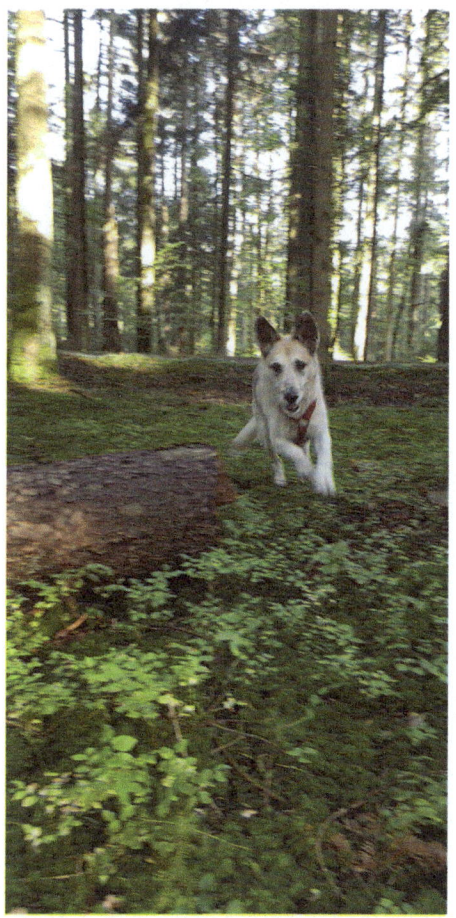

Sometimes new participants ask me where the dogs are housed outside of their deployment. Some mistakenly believe that therapy dogs live exclusively for their therapy deployment and live a completely different life than a "normal" family dog. I have therefore gotten into the habit of mentioning this self-evident fact, namely that the dogs live with me and are part of my family, always at the beginning of the therapy. This serves to sensitize the participant early on that therapy dogs are just normal dogs who want to live a dog-appropriate, beautiful life.

Beyond this *fundamental sense of security* (see Fig. 3.7), there are other aspects relevant for a dog's balanced private life. The term "balance" simply means to build a counterweight to something in order to achieve a healthy equilibrium. Therefore, the dog should receive offers from us in his leisure time that form a counterweight to what he experiences during therapy. What exactly these offers look like depends on what the dog does and experiences in therapy. This is similar to the breaks.

Fig. 3.6 Relaxed break with a nap

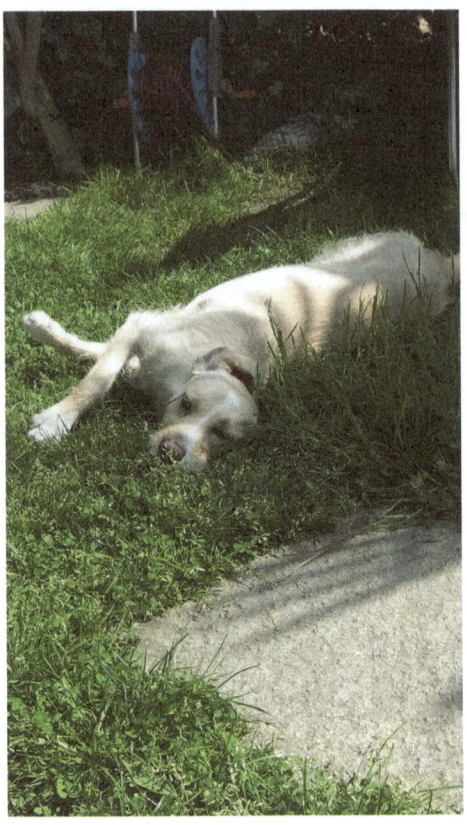

Since therapies are usually associated with various encounters and impressions for the dog and often take place in enclosed areas (be it a room or a fenced training area), *being able to move freely in nature* is a central aspect for a healthy balance. This means, for example, taking a quiet walk in the forest. It is good to let the dog be alone and at peace. Sniffing through the forest, stopping now and then, trotting a bit ahead, looking back, dawdling—this is the highest pleasure for dogs (see Fig. 3.8).

Studies have proven that being in the forest is beneficial for humans, as it significantly reduces stress (Hunter et al., 2019). In my experience, the same applies to dogs: In the forest, every dog feels like a small or large wolf; different areas of the brain are addressed and activated than when interacting with us humans. And this means primarily mental peace and relaxation for the dog. Allowing him these forest walks, as much as possible without commands,[2] is a great balance for the dog. Those who do not have

---

[2] This explicitly does not mean that the dog can disturb other walkers or wildlife as he likes. It goes without saying that we set a framework for the dog—calling him to us when we encounter walkers and of course not letting him chase or stir up wildlife. Within this framework, he can then move freely, i.e., without unnecessary speech and commands.

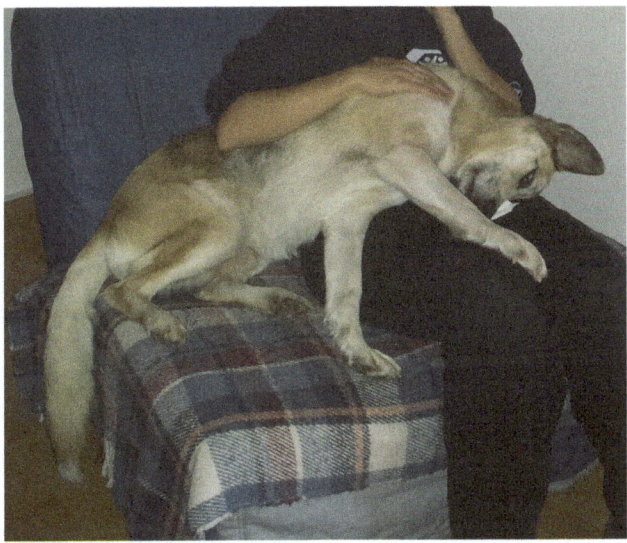

Fig. 3.7 Sense of security

a forest nearby can of course also use fields, meadows or other walking opportunities for the daily breaks and allow the dog undisturbed sniffing and exploration phases in between. In this case, I still recommend occasional trips to a forest area. The dog will greatly appreciate these, and it can be observed how tiring—in a positive sense—an extensive forest walk is for most dogs.

Another universally applicable aspect of creating a healthy balance is the *ability to play and be silly*. However, playing does not necessarily mean fetching. Because, when you sometimes observe dog-human pairs in everyday life, ball fetching sometimes seems to be more of a duty than a game for the dog. This can be seen when the dog would rather break out of the throw-fetch sequence or has to be called to bring the ball back. This does not mean that you should not practice fetching in this case—on the contrary, it can be a useful training. Especially for a pure family dog, who has no or few tasks to fulfill in everyday life, it can be useful to teach him to fetch.[3] What is meant here, however, is rather that if a dog is in therapy use and is not a big fan of bringing back when fetching, this exercise is not necessarily suitable as a playful balance. Because the game should mean exuberance and a balance to his training and his work for the dog.

---

[3] However, it is important to ensure that the dog has a basic interest in chasing and taking something into its mouth. Some dogs, depending on their disposition, have no ambitions for this and only look at their humans questioningly when they enthusiastically throw a ball for them. In this case, the saying "You can't carry a dog to the hunt" is very apt and one should resort to other exercises.

Fig. 3.8 Balance in the forest—Giulio on a discovery tour in the undergrowth

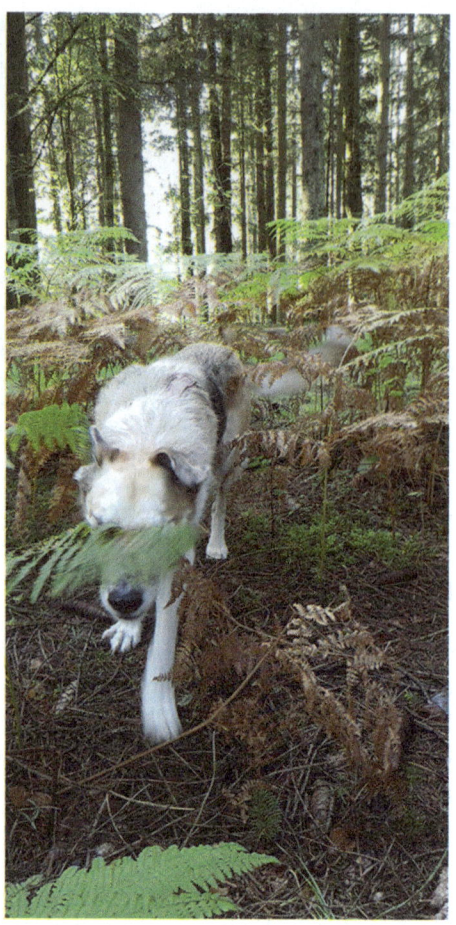

The game should therefore not be determined by us because we think, for example, that fetching in general is something great, but should be based on the individual character of the dog. For Cleo, for example, rolling on the grass and playful fighting with me are the most beautiful types of play (see Fig. 3.9). Giulio and Toni, on the other hand, are wilder and more diverse: They like to wrestle with each other and with their mistress, chase each other. Toni also likes to fetch (see Fig. 3.10). When Giulio has had a strenuous day, he loves to play powerfully and wrestle around a stick.

It is important to know what each dog experiences as a game and in which type of play he can be exuberant and funny. As mentioned, this varies greatly from dog to dog.

In addition to play, a healthy balance includes being *petted by a caregiver*. It makes a big difference to the dog whether it is petted during therapy by a participant or at home by its caregiver. Dogs, as mentioned, pick up on the emotions of the participants (see Silva & de Sousa, 2011; Sundman et al., 2019; Yong & Ruffman, 2014). In a therapy

Fig. 3.9 Cleo in her favorite game—rolling and fighting

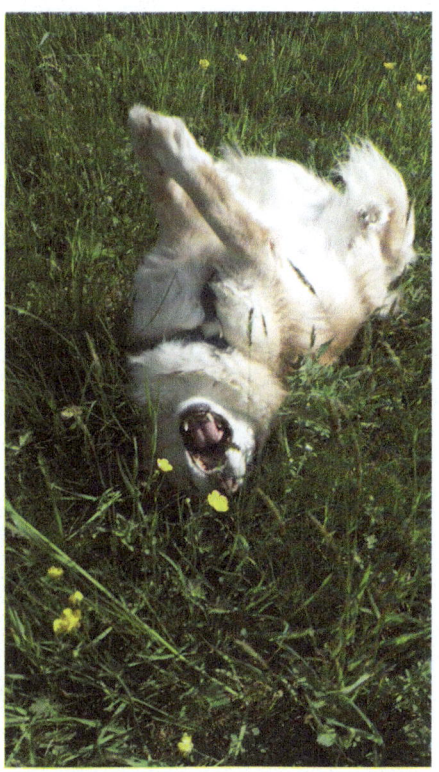

setting, these emotions are not always the most pleasant, but often fear, sadness, or tension. After therapy, a balance should be created by petting the dog in a particularly calming and relaxing way. Here, I recommend familiarizing yourself with common massage techniques (Mühlbauer, 2019). Even small tricks and tips can turn petting the dog into a relaxation procedure (see Fig. 3.11).

However, more important than the technique is the emotional state of the person petting. If we want the dog to relax through our petting, we should make sure to be as calm and relaxed as possible ourselves. The more relaxed we start petting the dog, the faster the dog relaxes, and this in turn also promotes our own relaxation. So, by petting the dog mindfully and relaxed, we are doing something good for both the dog and ourselves.

And finally, one last universally valid aspect for the important creation of a healthy balance for the dog: a *regular daily routine*. Dogs appreciate it when daily events happen at the same time. This creates predictability and thus security. It is good for the dog to have a daily rhythm, i.e., to eat, walk, work, and have leisure time at the same time. Of course, deviations are also part of this, and an appointment can cause the dog to eat later than usual, for example. Nevertheless, in general, the daily routine should have a regularity that is understandable for the dog.

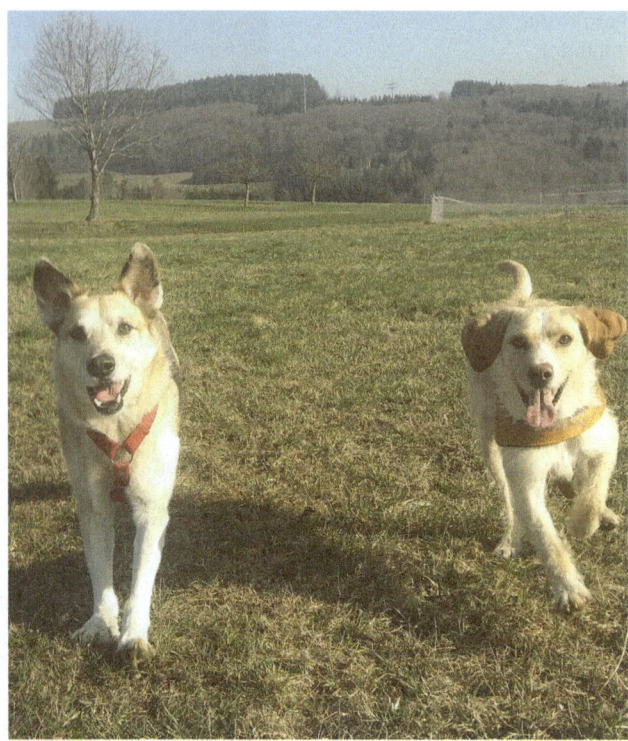

Fig. 3.10 Giulio and Toni frolicking

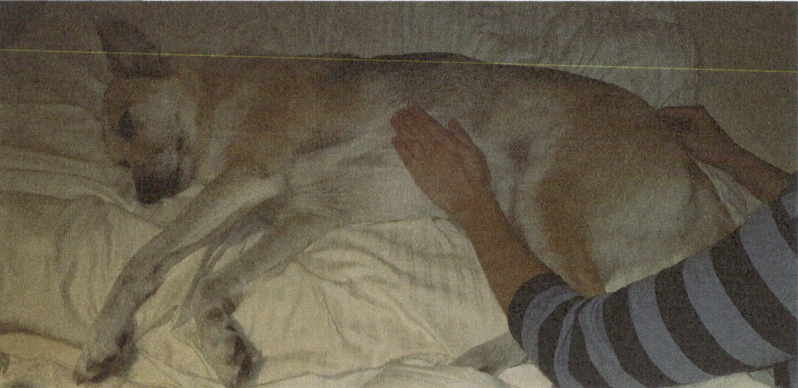

Fig. 3.11 Massage

When properly planning and carrying out breaks and compensatory activities for the dog, the therapist automatically reflects on the dog's working day. Is the volume of therapies currently high? How do the moods of the various participants affect the dog? How is the dog doing at the end of a deployment? Does he have the necessary joy in his work as a therapy support dog? The therapist asks questions concerning the dog and the therapies, which are important in order to be able to design sufficient and high-quality breaks and to create the right balance for the dog in his free time. The therapy content, the work processes, questioning one's own actions and oneself are closely related to this and, as further explained, are an important skill that a therapist working with animals should develop.

Summary: General Aspects for Creating a Healthy Balance for Dogs in Everyday Life:

- Foundation: the dog should feel unconditional love and security in its family
- In addition, it applies: The dog …
  - … needs duty-free times—so extensive walks, where he can walk and sniff at his own pace (ideally in the forest),
  - … must be allowed to play according to his taste—so play in a way that he can be exuberant (play in this sense should not become training!),
  - … benefits particularly from mindful and relaxing petting by his reference person,
  - … needs a daily rhythm (fixed feeding times, regulated times for feeding, walks, leisure, work and training).

3.8   Willingness to Self-Criticize

Who likes to question themselves? Probably no one. However, it is particularly important for animal-assisted therapists to do this regularly and consistently. Because in this area, you bear responsibility not only for yourself but also for the therapy participants and, above all, for the animals with which you work. And because the animals cannot speak up and say: "I'm not feeling so well today, I'd rather stay at home" or "I've always enjoyed jumping over obstacles, but lately my hip hurts, and I'd rather not do it so often", we as therapists bear a special responsibility (see Sect. 3.1).

Are the exercises we do in therapy suitable for the dog? Does he go to work with joy? Does he perhaps have complaints that are not visible at first glance? In general: What is good for the dog today may not be good tomorrow. So we may have designed the therapy to the best of our knowledge and belief to be suitable for dogs, and yet suddenly notice that the dog (perhaps due to age or health reasons, perhaps due to overload from years of patient contact) no longer enjoys the work. What to do in such a case? First, it is necessary to question whether it is the work itself or certain aspects of the work. If the latter is the case, then changing the working conditions can solve the problem. For example, a dog may have always enjoyed going to group therapy and then shows signs that he no longer wants to or can tolerate it. Early signs can be:

- reduced joy on the way there and when entering the building or premises,
- increased seeking of his resting place during the session,
- increased distance to the participants,
- or intense dreaming following days with this group session.

In an already advanced case, we see signs of stress in the dog before, during or after the session, recognizable for example by an increased occurrence of appeasement signals. A possible solution would be to conduct individual sessions with the dog instead of group therapies. However, it is again necessary to carefully check and critically question whether it is really only due to the number of participants, or whether the dog generally perceives his use as a therapy companion dog as stressful. Then it is time to end his deployment and send the dog into his well-deserved retirement—as painful and drastic as this decision may be for the human.

3.9   Knowing When It's Enough: Retirement

Retirement—this means that the dog no longer works as a therapy companion dog and continues to live in its family. This should be a matter of course. Firstly, because of the close relationship that exists between the therapist and his dog, but also because of the obligation towards the dog, who has faithfully served people for years. Unfortunately, it still happens that dogs, who have dedicated their best years to serving people, end up in animal shelters at the end of their lives. There are no exact figures for this and it is not the rule. Nevertheless, for example, some retired police dogs end up in animal shelters. Most police dogs stay with their handler after leaving service or are placed in families. But it happens that dogs, who have worked hard for people, receive no thanks or appreciation in the last phase of their lives. A sad and unfair circumstance. Therefore, at this point, the emphasis: A retired therapy companion dog stays in its family.

Considering this, in this section we will understand when the retirement of a therapy companion dog should begin and how it should be implemented.

3.9.1   When Should the Dog Retire?

At what point should a therapy companion dog retire? There is no fixed age limit for this, as every dog ages differently. One dog is still fit at thirteen years old and enjoys its work. Another dog is tired at eight years old and doesn't want to work anymore. It is therefore necessary to pay attention to certain signs in the dog to decide when it is time for him to retire.

Firstly, attention should be paid to the physical constitution of the dog. If *age-related physical limitations* occur, such as difficulties in walking or getting up, impaired vision or hearing, then the dog's retirement should be planned or at least prepared. The dog may not really seem restricted by these physical changes, as he can usually still manage his normal dog's day without any problems. However, due to these physical changes and limitations, the dog has to expend more energy to compensate for them. He should then no longer have to fulfill the additionally strenuous role of a therapy companion dog, which demands him emotionally and physically. The same applies to *age-independent chronic diseases* that restrict him and can affect dogs of any age. Here too, the dog should be allowed to retire. Another reason for starting retirement is when we notice that the *dog is therapy-tired*; that is, he loses his enjoyment of work, is emotionally overwhelmed or simply tired of the activity.

It is a difficult step to send your dog into retirement. Even though it is a matter of course that the dog then continues to live with us and remains part of the family, we as therapists lose our most beloved and important colleague at work. Making this decision is by no means trivial, but usually means a significant cut in the lives of all involved. Nevertheless, the highest commandment here too is the perception of our responsibility towards our dog in the sense of securing his well-being. For the therapist, it may be easier to let the dog work a little longer than is justifiable. But this motive must not be acted upon. The well-being of the dog must always and always be at the top, even if this may be associated with painful change, financial losses or other difficulties for us.

▶   **Important!** When deciding to retire the therapy companion dog, the well-being of the dog must always and always be at the top, even if this may be associated with painful change, financial losses or other difficulties for us.

3.9.2   How Do I Design the Path to Retirement?

Retirement means that the dog stays at home. Sometimes I see very old or therapy-tired dogs still being taken to therapies, simply to "be there". However, we must be aware that a dog, even if it does not perform exercises or the like, still absorbs the moods of the participants and has to process them. Therefore, I advocate not taking a retired therapy companion dog with you anymore, but leaving it at home in its familiar, family environment. Most dogs feel obliged to interact, to comfort, to offer themselves for petting, as soon as they are in the usual therapy setting due to their training and years of service. So they continue to work, even if it is not directly demanded of them.

Since suddenly staying at home is a big change for the dog, the retirement should be a slow gradual process. It is not advisable to simply stop taking the dog to work from one day to the next. Exceptions to this are situations of sudden illness or other unforeseen events that force an abrupt exit of the dog. As a rule and, if at all possible, we should prepare our dog's retirement slowly and design it as a gentle transition.

We start by slowly reducing his deployments, occasionally leaving him at home while we go to work with our other dog (Sect. 3.2). Here begins a reorientation process for all involved. It is important not to be disturbed by the initial behavior of the dog or to transfer our perhaps secret wish to continue working with our beloved dog onto the dog. Of course, he will want to go to work at the beginning. However, this behavior should not be misinterpreted so that one believes he absolutely wants to continue working. The dog is simply used to his previous daily rhythm. So if we, for example, get ready for work and leave, a "to-be-retired" dog naturally wants to continue to go along as usual in the first few days. But he does not want to go because he absolutely wants to continue working, but he simply wants to go because he has always gone along and that was his life. He must first learn that it can be different, that he can stay comfortably at home while mom or dad leave the house and go to work with the other dog. If we design this calmly, slowly and—very important—while maintaining all other beautiful leisure activities for the dog (Sect. 3.7), most dogs gratefully accept their retirement after a short time.

As therapists, we must therefore pay particular attention to the topic of retirement not to unconsciously transfer our wishes and needs onto the dog. If we perceive it as a painful cut not to be able to use and take the dog anymore, then we should deal with this feeling ourselves and independently consider the needs of the dog and not be guided by misinterpretations of his behavior. As mentioned, even an old or sick or therapy-tired dog has to get used to not working anymore—and, as we as dog experts know, any change is initially difficult for a dog. Hence we as humans have to take responsibility and, if necessary, slow him down and allow and gradually teach him to be "just" a family dog.

▶   **Important!** When retiring the therapy companion dog, it is important for the therapist to be careful not to unconsciously transfer his own wishes and needs onto the dog. Instead, it is necessary to take responsibility for the dog and allow and actively teach him to be just a family dog from now on.

As therapists, it should be our duty and satisfaction to see how our dog enjoys his retirement after possibly years of service. Retirement is as much a part of a therapy companion dog's life as the years of his training and the years of his work. It is to be wished and hoped that every dog, who has devoted a large part of his life to the service of people, can spend many healthy and happy years after his retirement.

The health of the dog is not always in our hands. However, we can and must do our part to enable our dog to enjoy his well-deserved retirement and make it as pleasant as possible for him. Nothing is worse for a dog than feeling like they no longer belong to the pack or are no longer important. The retired dog should not have to work anymore, but, as far as his constitution allows, should of course continue to participate in all the beautiful leisure activities (see Fig. 3.12).

Fig. 3.12 Retired but still involved—Cleo in the backpack

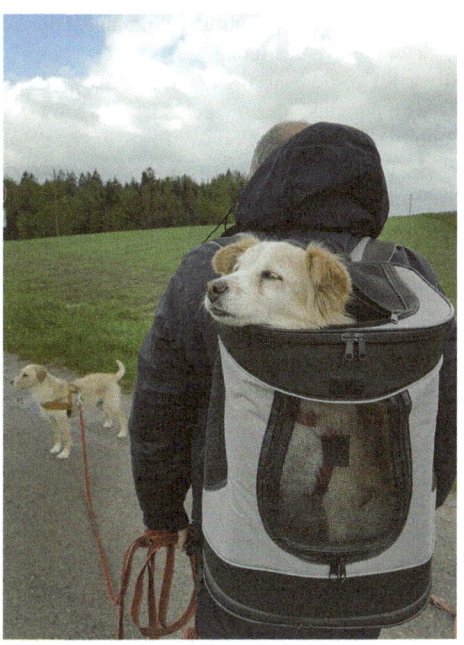

References

Blesch, K. (2013). *Hunde—Musik—Emotionen. Ein empirischer Vergleich der Wirkung von tierg-estützter und musiktherapeutischer Aktivität*. AV Akademiker.

Breeding Business. (2018). www.breedingbusiness.com/are-mixed-breed-dogs-healthier/. Accessed: 24. Oct. 2019.

Coppinger, R., & Coppinger, L. (2013). Hunde—Neue Erkenntnisse über Herkunft, Verhalten und Evolution der Kaniden. animal learn Verlag. www.animal-learn.de.

Coren, S. (1997). *Die Intelligenz der Hunde*. Rowohlt Taschenbuch.

Hunter, M. C. R., Gillespie, B. W., & Yu-Pu Chen, S. (2019). Urban nature experience reduce stress in the context of daily life based on salivary biomarkers. *Frontiers in Psychology, 10,* 722. https://doi.org/10.3389/fpsyg.2019.00722.

Marshall-Pescini, S., Frazzi, C., & Valsecchi, P. (2016). The effect of training and breed group on problem-solving behaviours of dogs. *Animal Cognition, 19*(3), 571–579.

Mehrkam, L., & Wynne, C. D. L. (2014). Behavioral differences among breeds of domestic dogs (canis lupus familiaris): Current status of science. *Applied Animal Behavior Science, 155,* 12–27.

Mühlbauer, B. (2019). *Hunde richtig massieren. Akupressur, Reflexzonen-Massage, TTouch und mehr*. Cadmos.

O'Neill, D. O., Church, D. B., McGreevy, P. D., Thomson, P. C., & Brodbelt, D. C. (2014). Prevalence of disorders recorded in dogs attending primary-care veterinary practices in England. *PLoS ONE, 9*(3), e90501. https://doi.org/10.1371/journal.pone.0090501.

Peta. (2013). https://www.peta.de/rassenwahn. Accessed: 9. Aug. 2019.

Reportagen. (2019). www.reportagen.de/reportagen/view/445/Tierquaelerei-fuer-einen-guten-Zweck. Accessed: 26. July 2019.

Rugaas, T. (2001). Calming Signals—Die Beschwichtigungssignale der Hunde. animal learn. www.animal-learn.de.

Silva, K., & de Sousa, L. (2011). Canis empathicus? A proposal on dogs' capacity to empathize with humans. *Biology Letters, 7,* 489–492.

Sundman, A. S., Van Poucke, E., Svensson Holm, A. C., Faresjö, A., Theodorsson, E., & Roth, L. S. (2019). Long-term stress levels are synchronized in dogs and their owners. *Scientific Report, 9*(7391), 1–7.

Switzer, E., & Nolte, I. (2007). Ist der Mischling wirklich der gesündere Hund? Untersuchung zur Erkrankungsanfälligkeit bei Mischlingen in Deutschland. *Praktischer Tierarzt, 88*(1), 14–19.

Yong, M. H., & Ruffman, T. (2014). Emotional contagion: Dogs and humans show a similar physiological response to human infant crying. *Behavioural Processes, 108,* 155–165.

Animal-Assisted Therapy with Dogs from Animal Welfare—Limits and Opportunities

4

Contents

Abstract

In the previous chapters, I have explained why the use of dogs from animal shelters is ethically commendable and what to consider for a dog-friendly animal-assisted therapy. In this chapter, I would like to explain the specific characteristics a future therapy companion dog should have. The next step is about how to assess a dog from an animal shelter in terms of its character and thus its suitability for therapeutic work. Furthermore, the special opportunities of animal-assisted work with dogs from animal shelters are explained. Finally, the challenges of training shelter dogs are also highlighted.

K. Blesch, *Animal-Assisted Therapy with Dogs*,
https://doi.org/10.1007/978-3-662-67965-4_4

4.1   Necessary Characteristics of a (Future) Therapy Dog

It is still common to use dogs in therapy that come from breeding. Certain breeds are described by breeders or sometimes by associations as particularly suitable for use in therapy. The practitioner, who may be planning his first steps in animal-assisted therapy, is given the impression that he can only get a foothold in therapy if he acquires a suitable dog. This is the case because it is often implied that a therapy dog must meet certain external criteria such as: The dog should come from a breeder and belong to a certain breed. Or the dog should start preparing for his later work as a therapy dog as a puppy. Since such criteria cannot usually be met by dogs that come from animal welfare or animal shelters, it is often an unwritten rule in the animal-assisted therapy industry that rescue animals are not suitable for use in therapy.

However, if one analyzes which characteristics are actually relevant and necessary, it becomes clear that dogs from animal welfare can be just as suitable for use in therapy as dogs from breeding. Because it is exclusively characteristics that concern the nature of the dog that determine whether he is suitable as a therapy dog or not.

Specifically, in my experience, the important and fundamental characteristics of a therapy dog concern neither his appearance nor his pedigree, but rather his *character* and his *reactions*.

> ▶   **Important!** A dog is suitable as a therapy dog due to character traits—not
>   because of his appearance or origin.

The character of a therapy dog should be characterized by *openness*, *friendliness* and *sociability* towards humans. Therapy dogs should therefore meet new people with interest and openness. They should show friendly behaviors during interaction with humans and generally enjoy contact with humans. The dog should bring these characteristics with him. It is also self-evident that the behavior and reactions of the human also play a role. If a person approaches the dog in a friendly to neutral manner, then the aforementioned should apply and the dog should show open, friendly behavior. However, if a person is unfriendly, harsh or disrespectful to the dog, then it should be clear that the openness and friendliness of the dog also has and must have limits.

And this leads to the second central characteristic of a therapy dog, namely his reactions to stressors. Here, the dog should neither be easily frightened nor should he show aggressive behavior. Rather, he should be able to *deal with stressors confidently*. Stressors are external events that cause stress in the dog. Such events in the context of therapy can be certain human behaviors that are unpleasant to the dog, or occurrences in the environment. A realistic stressor in the context of animal-assisted therapy would be, for example, a patient speaking loudly or shouting. The dog may and should indeed show that he finds the volume unpleasant. Especially for people who tend to be impulsive, it can be an important learning experience to realize that the loud voice is perceived as threatening by the other person. The dog may then react with distance, for example by lying down in his retreat place or going to the therapist. However, it is important that the dog does not react to such behaviors with fear or aggressive behavior.

Another realistic example is a sudden loud noise like a falling object or a siren. Of course, the dog may flinch in such a case, just like we humans do when a sudden loud noise surprises us. But beyond that, the dog should not show a fear reaction.

By meeting these two important criteria regarding character and reaction, a dog brings the basic prerequisites for its use in therapy. This makes it a pleasant interaction partner for its human counterpart, poses no danger or risk, and can even enjoy the therapy itself, as it fundamentally likes contact with humans. I would like to remind you at this point that the joy and well-being of the dog in therapy also crucially depends on the design of the therapy and the living conditions allowed for the dog (see Sect. 3.4). In the following section, I will explain how to determine whether the dog meets the described criteria regarding its character and reactions.

4.2   Assessment of Suitability as a Therapy Dog

Many of the concerns about adopting a dog from an animal shelter, and especially about its use in animal-assisted therapy, are related to the worry of not being able to assess a dog from an animal shelter. One thought might be: One does not know what the dog has exactly experienced, so one cannot estimate whether it might be reminded of a traumatic situation at some point and then bite.

It is true that we can never know exactly what a dog from an animal shelter has experienced before its time with us. However, to assess its character and reactions to stressors, and thus to assess its potential as a therapy dog, we do not need to know this.

When we get to know a dog from an animal shelter and wonder if it is suitable as a therapy dog, two possibilities arise:

- The dog has the necessary characteristics of a therapy dog
- The dog does *not* have the necessary characteristics of a therapy dog

A truly traumatized dog will always fall into the second category, as it is a dog characterized by increased alertness, mistrust of new and unfamiliar things, and strong reactions to threatening situations. A traumatized dog thus cannot meet the criteria of *open, friendly, sociable character* and especially *sovereign reactions to stressors*. If we pay attention to these criteria, there is no realistic danger that the dog we choose would be traumatized or unpredictable.

So how do we check the dog's basic character and reactions in contact with it? I recommend anyone who does not have specific training in this area and also does not have extensive experience with dogs to seek knowledgeable guidance and advice when choosing a dog from a shelter or animal rescue, for example from a reputable dog trainer. Nev-

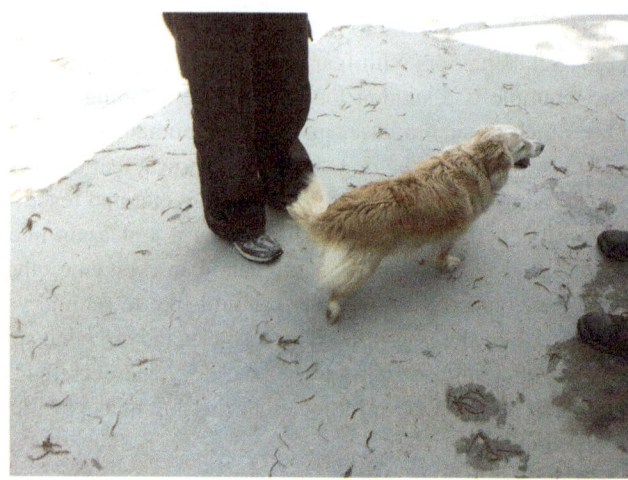

Fig. 4.1 First meeting with Cleo at the animal shelter—Cleo meets us openly, friendly, and without fear

ertheless, for orientation I would like to briefly mention how the character and reactions of a dog can be assessed.

▶   **Important!** Anyone who does not have a solid training and reliable experience in dealing with dogs from animal shelters should seek support from a professional when choosing a dog from a shelter.

Firstly, it is important to observe the dog attentively during our initial contact and to pay attention to the criteria for sociability and openness during the first contact listed in the checklist (see Fig. 4.1). Furthermore, we observe how the dog approaches or reacts to other people. It is good to see him interacting with different people (i.e., with women, men, and children).[1] After we have checked openness and sociability during the initial contact, we look at the dog's friendliness in different interactions and situations in the second step. Especially during play, the dog can still be boisterous, but it is important that he remains friendly at all times.

The next, more difficult step is then to assess the dog's reactions to stressors. This requires experience—both experience with dogs and professional experience as an animal-assisted therapist. If this experience is not available, expert support should be sought at this point at the latest. The aim now is to check how the dog deals with stress-inducing

---

[1] It may be that dogs react reservedly or shyly to groups of people they do not know. For example, if dogs see a person in a wheelchair or with a walking aid, or someone with a different skin color for the first time, their openness may be limited. However, if we know that the dog is open and friendly to us and other people, usually only introduction and habituation are needed here.

events that may occur in therapy. The clearer it already is with which clientele and in which setting the dog will work in the future, the more specifically potential stressors can be identified and the dog can be confronted with them.

However, it is generally important at this point that it is not about anticipating and trying out all possible therapy settings and experiences. This is part of the later training and is not relevant at this point. The goal is to assess how the dog reacts to stressors and to rule out that he shows strong fear reactions or aggressive behavior. It is solely about assessing his basic suitability as a therapy dog. At this point, the dog will not yet know and be able to do many things—this should be clear. We only want to check here how he reacts when he is unsettled by situations or behaviors that are unpleasant for a dog. If he reacts calmly or with a brief fright, calms down immediately afterwards and remains curious in contact with us, then this is healthy, confident dog behavior and thus a positive confirmation of his suitability for use as a therapy dog. If, on the other hand, the dog reacts fearfully, suspiciously or even defensively-aggressively beyond a brief moment of fright, then this is an indicator that this dog should not be used for therapy.

Checklist for Assessing a Dog's Character and Reactions
- In the initial contact with us and other people, the dog shows openness and sociability by…:
  - … initiating contact or approaching on its own,
  - … moving without hesitation,
  - … reacting with interest,
  - … making eye contact with a soft, benevolent expression in its eyes,
  - … seeking closeness,
  - … indicating that it wants to be petted (for example, by nudging or leaning).
- In further encounters, the dog's friendliness is expressed by…:
  - … allowing itself to be touched without any problems,
  - … being benevolent and friendly while playing and romping,
  - … allowing things to be taken from its mouth,
  - … running and jumping during joint runs, but not snapping,
  - … allowing itself to be slowed down if it plays too boisterously,
  - … reacting friendly and interested when the person sits down on the ground next to it,
  - … dealing with everyday situations, such as being fed or leashed, without any problems.
- When the dog is further confronted with stressors, it reacts without fear or aggressive behavior to:[2]

---

[2]The dog may flinch briefly at sudden noises. This is a natural reaction. However, it should not show any further fear reaction. It may also show that these situations are unpleasant for it, for example by calmly keeping a greater distance from the noise source. But this must be done without signs of fear or aggression.

- loud shouting or screaming,
- clattering with objects,
- quick, sudden gesticulating,
- being hugged and briefly held,
- being in a small space with several people.

As mentioned, we do not have a fully trained therapy dog in our hands just because this dog has the necessary basic characteristics of a therapy dog. We merely have good prerequisites to work with and train him. From here, a lot can still go wrong, but this now depends on our skills and abilities in dealing with dogs. As the saying goes, the responsibility for the dog's behavior is to be found *at the other end of the leash*, that is, in the hands of the human.

A friendly, open, sociable dog that is confident in dealing with stressors is not a guarantee. If a person has such a dog by his side, it is now his responsibility for the further positive development of the dog. This applies equally to dogs that come from breeding or animal protection. From the moment the person brings the dog home, the responsibility for the dog's further development lies solely in the hands of the human.

4.3   Special Opportunities of Working with a Therapy Dog from Animal Protection

In my experience, therapy dogs from animal protection are characterized not only by their individual character traits but also by a high sensitivity to human moods, gratitude, and a more or less pronounced ability to be autonomous.

4.3.1   High Sensitivity to Human Moods

In animal welfare, two broad categories of dogs can be distinguished: stray dogs and surrendered family dogs. Both types of dogs have usually experienced changing caregivers and in this context had to develop a pronounced sensitivity to human moods.

For a dog that started life as a family dog and was then surrendered, it can be assumed that before his surrender, he usually experienced at least two different living conditions and caregivers. Namely: The people in the environment where he was born and spent the first weeks, and the people and the home where he lived until his surrender. In the animal shelter, he then continues to meet changing caregivers and volunteers.

The surrender from home and the admission to the animal shelter are also emotional events—primarily, of course, for the affected dog, but also for the involved people. There may have been disputes in the family beforehand. A family member may have developed an allergy and the family surrenders the dog with great sadness. The owner may have died. The dog may have experienced rejection from some family members; there may have been anger and aggression. In short, there can be various motives and thus emotions that lead to the surrender of a dog. Only one thing is quite clear: the surrender of a dog to an animal shelter rarely happens completely emotionless and sober; emotions are usually involved.

For a dog that has lived part of his life on the street, the number of changing interactions with humans is even higher. At the same time, the existential relevance of interactions with humans is higher. Is the person approaching the dozing dog a dog lover bringing food, or does he want to chase the dog away? Are the teenagers a threat to the dog or do they want to play with him? Who is dangerous, who is friendly? Who approaches the dog with tension and contempt? Who with a loving smile and a few bites of food? Who smells of fear? Who might kick the dog? Who is friendly, who is neutral? Street dogs must be able to quickly and reliably assess people, otherwise their health and survival are concretely endangered.

If a dog—whether after surrender or after a life as a stray dog—then lives a little longer in the animal shelter, he also experiences different moods with different people here. One caregiver will always be loving and attentive to the dog; another caregiver will be more patient or more stressed depending on the day's constitution. The next caregiver may always behave distantly to the dog.[3] The dogs in the shelter experience only a few stimuli from the outside, and each of these stimuli (feeding, cleaning the box, exercise, walk) is associated with a human interaction. Also, in southern countries like Italy, shelter changes are not uncommon. To increase a dog's chances of adoption, he is moved to another shelter or sometimes brought to another country by animal welfare organizations. These changes are also a challenge for the dog, as he now has to adjust to a new environment, a stress-laden journey, and again to new people.

Thus, a dog in the setting of the animal shelter quickly learns to assess people and to perceive their moods early on. Especially when people come to take the dog for a walk or even to choose for adoption. A person walking through the corridors of the animal shelter looking for a dog that appeals to him will show sympathy, interest, displeasure, fear, and the like through his facial expressions. And dogs can read our facial expressions better than is often assumed (Albuquerque et al., 2016). The animal shelter is therefore a place where dogs develop an even better ability to quickly read human emotions due to the high importance of human moods for the dog.

Dogs from animal shelters usually have a high sensitivity to human moods due to the circumstances of their life before their arrival at the shelter and their time in the shelter. They have developed the ability to respond well to people and their moods. They are sen-

---

[3] For the caregivers' interaction with the dogs, it is certainly crucial, besides individual character traits, why someone works in the animal shelter, i.e. whether it is a job or whether caring for the dogs is also a matter of the heart for that person.

sitive and respond delicately to the atmosphere around them. If these dogs then meet the previously described suitability criteria (see Sect. 4.1), they are the most suitable dogs for use in therapy.

4.3.2   Gratitude

If you ask the new owners of dogs from animal shelters about the characteristics of their dog, "gratitude" will be one of the most frequently mentioned traits. Dogs that have been surrendered or abandoned to the shelter and may have experienced neglect, loneliness, and dreary living conditions, not only flourish when they are provided with a reliable and loving family life. They also know the contrast. They know what a bad life is. These dogs usually have a high level of gratitude towards their people.

Why is this good for therapy? There are two reasons:

Firstly, the therapist has a loyal colleague in a grateful dog. Of course, this does not mean that as a human, one should confuse this gratitude with subservience and exploit it in the sense of disregarding the dog's needs! A grateful dog is a loyal colleague in therapy and, if the therapist reciprocates this gratitude and loyalty of the dog with gratitude towards the dog, a wonderful human-dog team is formed. And the better the team, the better the therapeutic work.

The dog's gratitude also has another effect on therapy. The dog's gratitude can be discussed with the participant, consciously perceived, and understood as an important resource in life. Those who are grateful are not bitter. Those who are grateful see the good that surrounds them. Those who are grateful have a benevolent view of themselves and life. Gratitude contradicts depressive or anxious thinking in many ways. Thus, there are various therapeutic approaches that consciously aim at developing the feeling of gratitude, such as concepts of positive psychology. And with the presence of a dog that truly lives the attitude of gratitude, this feeling can be well developed and promoted in the participant.

4.3.3   Possibility of Identification for Patients

Those who experience mental suffering, those who seek therapeutic help, are overall or in parts not doing well in life—and often for quite a long time. Many participants can therefore identify well with a dog that has had to experience bad things in life, who knows what loneliness and abandonment feel like or has had to make other experiences of disregard. The story of the dog's previous life circumstances often resonates with the participant, evoking an empathetic feeling of understanding and familiarity.

And this forms the basis for various therapeutic interventions. The feeling of identification with the dog can, for example, be used to introduce the concept of hope for change, which many participants lack. The situation of the dog (I personally refer here

Fig. 4.2 The dog looked stressed and unkempt in the shelter …

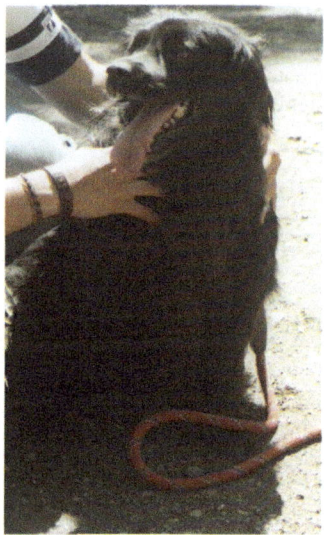

mostly to the life story of Giulio Sect. 1.3.2) seemed quite hopeless. Yet it could be overcome. A change in ingrained behaviors, believed to be impossible, was indeed possible. It required patience, practice, and a willingness to change—both from Giulio himself and from all his caregivers and from me, who trained and educated him.

In therapy, I sometimes introduce the image or idea to the participants of being a good coach to themselves in the therapy process, who lovingly and patiently enables change. If a part of the participant believes "I can't do this", then the image can be promoted that there are other parts inside the participant besides this fear. And one part can, for example, be a patient coach who encourages, believes in change, and does not give up.

Many participants no longer believe in actual change in their lives. Sometimes this is a symptom of a depressive illness, sometimes it is learned helplessness, lack of self-efficacy, or low self-confidence that prevent belief in the possibility of change. An important aspect of the therapeutic process is therefore to develop and strengthen the desire for change and the active hope for an improvement of things. The symbolic image of the dog, who despite all adversities was able to grow out of a seemingly hopeless situation, can be extremely helpful for this (see comparison between Fig. 4.2 and 4.3).

4.3.4 Feeling of Meaningfulness

Another special feature in working with a therapy dog from animal welfare is that dealing with them can be perceived as particularly meaningful by some participants.

In crises or during depressive episodes, those affected often experience activities as devoid of meaning. "What's the point of all this?" or "This won't make my life any bet-

Fig. 4.3 After his adoption, the dog physically and mentally blossomed—a significant change

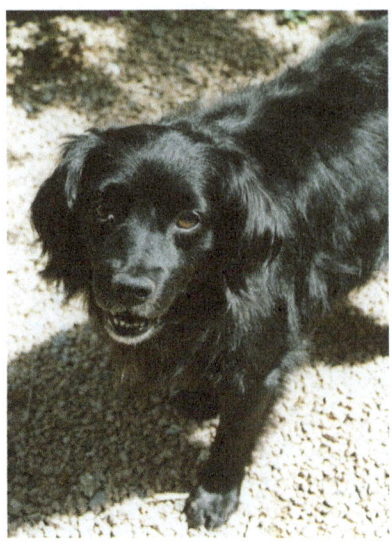

ter," are common statements that a therapist hears at the beginning of therapy. In relation to the discussions in group therapy, these could be remarks like "What good will it do me to listen to the problems of complete strangers?". However, the fact that listening, reporting personal experiences, and exchanging with other affected people can trigger internal processes and thus bring movement into hardened thought structures, is not (yet) apparent to those affected in such moments. The feeling of meaninglessness is a symptom of a depressive illness or depressive reaction to a life event and at the same time prevents or makes it difficult to engage in beneficial activities. Often it is a process, at the beginning of which initially stands the externally promoted overcoming, and in the course of which an internal engagement increasingly arises.

For some, it can help at the beginning to know that the dog also benefits from the therapy. Because his work as a therapy dog has given him the opportunity to leave the animal shelter or the street and lead a happy dog life. Only the work as a therapy dog (i.e., the work with the participant) gave the dog the chance to live a good life. Depending on individual attitudes, participants may like the idea of doing good. It gives them an additional feeling of meaningfulness in a phase when many things seem devoid of meaning, and facilitates engagement with the content of the therapy.

4.4 Challenges in Working with a Therapy Dog from Animal Welfare

Those who embark on new paths must not only look forward to pleasant things, but also automatically adjust to certain adversities. Thus, working with a dog from animal welfare not only brings much pleasure but also challenges. If one is aware of these challenges in advance and approaches them mindfully, they can be well mastered.

The selection of a suitable dog must be given the *necessary care and time*. Under no circumstances should one feel pressured by the duration of the search. It may well be that one has to look at several dogs in several animal shelters before finding "the right one". And at this point, it must also be mentioned that going to the animal shelter is rarely easy, as a dog lover feels touched by most dogs. Nevertheless, one should not make a compromise, i.e., take a dog that is only partially suitable. There is nothing more irresponsible than offering a dog a home at last and then surrender it again. The same applies if one is immediately enthusiastic about a dog and overlooks its lack of suitability as a therapy dog due to a feeling of enthusiasm.

Dogs that come from animal welfare can be *prematurely aged* or bring *physical complaints* due to previous poor nutritional conditions and lack of health care. Cleo, for example, has heart failure due to her severe illness, which she contracted during her time on the street. She requires regular check-ups and takes medicine to support her heart function. One must be aware of this: a dog that has lived a life in which he was not consistently well cared for can suffer certain physical complaints due to the consequences. These can be evident at the time of adoption or may only become apparent in old age. And of course, necessary veterinary treatments and medications cost money. Also, pre-existing conditions may mean that the dog does not live as long as he could have if he had lived a good life from the start. However, it should also be clear that there is never a guarantee of health or a long life—neither for dogs nor humans. A dog can have been raised and kept under the best conditions and still fall ill even at a young age.

Another aspect that makes working with a dog from an animal shelter more difficult—or I would rather say—more challenging, is the *training*. Often, the dogs are already a bit older, so they are no longer puppies, when one starts working with them. In addition, they may show behaviors that need to be unlearned. This can make the training and preparation for therapy use potentially a bit more protracted and demand more competencies from the trainer. Therefore, this aspect is dedicated to a separate chapter.

Last but not least, it should be emphasized at this point that animal-assisted work with dogs from animal shelters is not yet a matter of course. It is therefore quite possible that one may encounter *prejudices*, have to patiently explain or deal with criticism. For example, one may be directly or indirectly confronted with the prejudice that mixed breeds and shelter dogs are inferior dogs compared to certain purebred dogs. In this regard, I have found that such prejudices are best refuted by the dogs themselves. How often have I been asked by participants at the beginning of therapy or by colleagues what "special breed" Giulio is. People ask this because they experience what a fine and loving nature

Giulio has, and simply cannot imagine that "such a great dog" is a mixed breed and comes from an animal shelter.

Anyone now considering the path of combining animal welfare and therapy should be aware of the special challenges mentioned here in animal-assisted work with dogs from animal shelters and incorporate them into their decision.

Summary: Possible Stumbling Blocks in Working with a Therapy Companion Dog from an Animal Shelter:

- It *can* take time to find the suitable dog from an animal shelter, as the selection of the dog must be done carefully, based on sensible criteria (see Sect. 4.1) and with calmness
- A dog from an animal shelter *can* potentially be prematurely aged and have physical complaints
- The training of a dog from an animal shelter *can* be more demanding and take longer than the training of another dog
- One can be confronted with *prejudices* regarding shelter dogs

These points should be carefully considered and one should only decide on a dog from an animal shelter if one is willing to deal with these aspects.

Reference

Albuquerque, N., Guo, K., Wilkinson, A., & Savalli, C. (2016). Dogs recognize dog and human emotions. *Biology Letters, 12*(1), 20150883. https://doi.org/10.1098/rsbl..2015.0883.

The Dog-Assisted Self-Confidence Training

5

Contents

Supplementary Information The online version contains supplementary material available at https://doi.org/10.1007/978-3-662-67965-4_5. The videos can be accessed individually by clicking the DOI link in the accompanying figure caption or by scanning this link with the SN More Media App.

Abstract

In this chapter, I present a concept for a dog-assisted self-confidence training that I have developed and use for working with self-doubting individuals. First, I discuss general aspects of the target group as well as the duration and framework of the training, and then introduce the concept of self-confidence in the following section. Subsequent explanations are given as to why self-confidence can be trained so well with dogs, and how exactly self-confidence is expressed when dealing with a dog. Afterwards, I will introduce the specific course of the training using examples from practice. Finally, I will highlight possible difficulties in the course of the dog-assisted self-confidence training.

5.1   Framework and Background of Dog-Assisted Self-Confidence Training

The following section describes the framework and background of dog-assisted self-confidence training. It describes the target groups for the training, how long it lasts, and how it was developed. It then goes on to discuss self-confidence and why it can be well developed and promoted with dogs. Finally, this section clearly explains how dogs specifically react to self-confident and self-doubting behavior. This is relevant because the dogs' reactions to the participants' behavior form the basis for the self-confidence training.

5.1.1   Target Groups, Duration, and Origin

The target group for dog-assisted self-confidence training are individuals who suffer from their lack of self-confidence. Lack of self-confidence has a large overlap with mental illnesses and impairments. Without being able to delve into this topic at this point, examples of these overlaps are mentioned: In the context of a depressive illness, self-esteem, self-confidence, and self-efficacy are impaired. Those suffering from an anxiety disorder or phobia are situationally or generally self-doubting. Or, as a renowned professor of clinical psychology and psychotherapy puts it:

"Self-doubt and lack of self-confidence can be observed in a variety of mental disorders. (…) such as phobias, obsessive-compulsive disorders, depression" (Fiedler & Marwitz, 2016, p. 217).

Thus, building self-confidence is an aspect of treating mental illnesses, and the main target groups of dog-assisted self-confidence training are therefore people with mental impairments.

However, the training is not limited to these target groups. In the sense of prevention, other target groups are all those individuals who regularly perceive themselves as self-doubting. These could include, for example:

- Adolescents and young adults with insecure demeanor and/or insecurity in social situations
- Individuals who experience a major change, crises, or significant experiences and are therefore in a situation of general uncertainty

In addition, the self-confidence training promotes a person's general leadership competence and is therefore also suitable for individuals who hold a supervisory role in their profession and want to analyze or improve their individual leadership style.

Ultimately, self-confidence training can benefit many, if not most, people. Life, through changes and conflicts, continually tests self-confidence. Therefore, it can only be beneficial for most people to consciously promote and strengthen their own confidence from time to time. Studies also indicate how important self-confidence is for personal and professional satisfaction. For example, the authors around Campbell-Meiklejohn show in their study using imaging techniques that the human brain is set up to attribute more importance to the opinions of confident people (Campbell-Meiklejohn et al., 2017). At the same time, studies suggest that self-confidence can be well developed or increased in the context of training (see Lehenbauer, 2012 for this).

But as with any form of therapy, there are also contraindications for dog-assisted self-confidence training, i.e., cases in which it is advised against carrying out the training. Specifically, these contraindications concern individuals:

- who suffer from dog hair allergies,
- for whom the training with the dog would be too strenuous or risky due to severe physical impairments,
- who have shown animal cruelty in the past or clearly lack respect for animals,
- who suffer from mental illnesses with significant psychotic symptoms[1] .

The first two contraindications concern the integrity of the participant, the last two the integrity of the dog. Participation should be considered in cases of mild manifestations of psychotic symptoms. However, a prior clarification and close exchange with the treating psychotherapist or psychiatrist are recommended. It must be ensured that the participant does not show aggressive impulse breakthroughs that could endanger the dog. It must also be ensured that the participant is able to follow instructions during training with the dog. Then, even in the presence of psychotic symptoms, participation is possible—as said, after consultation with the therapists.

However, if individuals have shown animal cruelty or have no respect for animals, I consistently refrain from their participation in dog-assisted self-confidence training.

---

[1] In the context of psychotic symptoms, a person's thinking and perception are usually altered. Since the symptoms are diverse, they are not per se an exclusion criterion. Psychotic symptoms pose a risk to working with the dog when it can be assumed that impulse breakthroughs and aggressive behavior can occur as part of delusional symptoms.

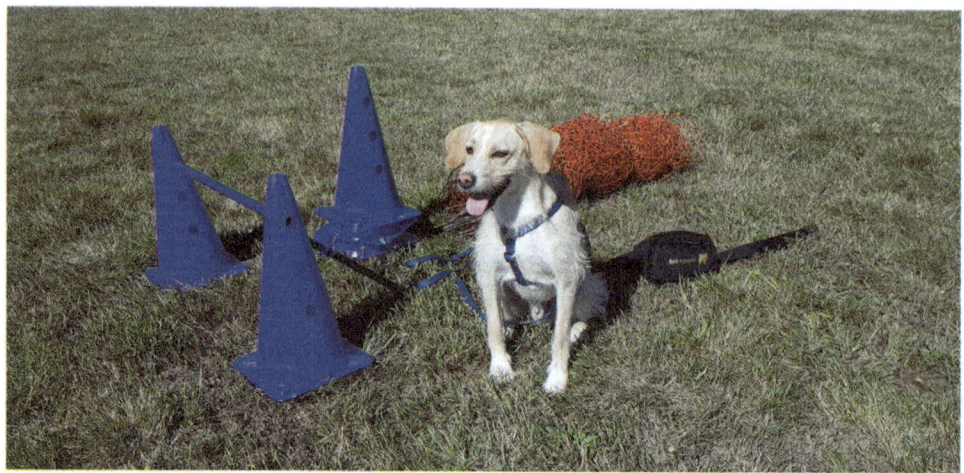

Fig. 5.1   Toni with harness, leash, pylons, bar, mobile sheep fence

Certainly, sadistic behavior often has a treatable disorder at its root. Nevertheless, this is not to be treated in this context, but in the context of psychotherapy. Supervised contact with animals should only be made possible for these individuals when the treatment has already borne its first fruits.

In any case, the physical and mental integrity and the general well-being of the dog or animal always come first. This aspect must be considered in every decision about a person's participation in dog-assisted self-confidence training.

I designed the dog-assisted self-confidence training for ten sessions. Of course, the duration can vary depending on the participant. The first session is for getting to know each other and for the initial conversation, the content of which will be explained in more detail below. This is followed by the practical training sessions, starting with the second session. In this session, the participant interacts spontaneously with the dog, which is especially important for my assessment of the participant's self-confidence. Based on this, I give the participant feedback on the external impact of their self-confidence. This feedback takes place at the end of the second or at the beginning of the third session. Based on this, I determine the exact focus of the self-confidence training together with the participant. In the following sessions, the participant practices leading the dog confidently with and without a leash, with progressively increasing difficulty and taking into account their individual focus. The last session, in addition to the final practical exercises with the dog, serves to summarize what has been learned in the context of a final discussion.

I have gathered experiences with the implementation of dog-assisted self-confidence training in clinics and private training sessions. I have been conducting this training since 2011 with my therapy dogs Giulio, Toni, and Cleo (more about the dogs in Sect. 1.3.2). Cleo has not been working since early 2019 due to age (more on the topic of retirement of a therapy dog in Sect. 3.9). Toni started actively participating as a therapy dog in self-confidence training during the same period after appropriate training. I started and developed the dog-assisted self-confidence training in private courses in Germany and Italy. As a form of therapy, I have been conducting it since 2012 in Germany, initially at a psychosomatic rehabilitation clinic and subsequently at a psychosomatic and psychiatric acute clinic, as well as with private participants.

The training can essentially be carried out anywhere. The following equipment or premises are required (see Fig. 5.1):

- for the dog
  - a comfortable harness and a standard leash, possibly an additional long leash,
  - tasty treats,
  - quiet and retreat opportunities,
  - a bowl with always fresh water,
- for the participant
  - an adjustable waist bag for the treats,
- in general
  - several pylons,
  - obstacles or a bar matching the pylons,
  - a mat,
  - a quiet room for pre- and post-discussion of the training sessions,
  - a secluded, quiet practice area of at least five by ten meters, which can be used alone with the participant and the dog.[2]

5.1.2   Self-confidence

The goal of dog-assisted self-confidence training is to increase self-confidence. The basis for my training is a concept of self-confidence that is inseparably linked with social competence and can be described as follows:

▶ **Definition: "Self-confidence"** "In interpersonal, social situations, a self-confident and socially competent person has humane, i.e., self- and other-appreciating, attitudes, value systems, basic assumptions, and planning structures. This person has in these situations a) the ability to encourage, appreciate, and respect themselves and others; b) courage, serenity, security, trust, and the ability to cope with impairments of these emotions; c) sufficient peace and relaxation, or the ability to allow impairments of physical reactions,

---

[2]If you want or need to be flexible here, use a sheep fence that can be easily set up and taken down.

and d) a wide range of appropriate, goal-oriented, and authentic behaviors and manners."
(Güroff, 2018, p. 25)

A prerequisite for the development of self-confidence is the feeling of *self-efficacy*. That
is, the feeling of being able to influence events and situations and generally being able to
impact one's own life.

Perceived self-efficacy and self-confidence are central foundations for a satisfied life.
Because: Those who have a sense of self-efficacy strive to actively shape their life and
relationships. Those who are self-confident have an appreciative relationship with themselves and their environment. Those who are self-confident have resources to deal with
adversities in the best possible way. Those who are self-confident dare to approach new
situations and challenges.

To distinguish from *self-confident* behavior are *self-insecure* and *aggressive* behavior.
I understand self-insecure and aggressive behavior as two sides of the same coin. One
side is the quiet, the other side the loud expression of inner insecurity. One strategy is
to withdraw into oneself to protect one's perceived vulnerability. The other strategy is to
protect one's perceived vulnerability through a dominant appearance.

▶   **Important!** Self-insecure and aggressive behavior are to be understood as two
     sides of the same coin and as the opposite pole to self-confident behavior.

We recognize the common root of the two behaviors also in that they often merge into
each other or condition each other. Consider, for example, passive-aggressive behavior,
where inner aggressions only timidly emerge outward. Or the famous outbursts of anger
after long "swallowing" and pent-up negative emotions. Or embarrassed, insecure behavior after an outburst of anger. In all these situations, aggression and insecurity go hand in
hand.

Example: Transition from self-insecure to aggressive behavior

An employee repeatedly agrees to perform additional tasks—not out of conviction or
enjoyment of the activity, but out of fear of saying no to the supervisor. He is annoyed
about it, but shows adapted behavior outwardly. Perhaps he also tries to get out of the
situation by looking for excuses ("I am not suitable for this"), but without confidently
representing his view. At some point, he is asked again to perform an additional task
and instead of confidently saying no, all the pent-up anger bursts out of him in a fit of
rage. This is a possible example of how self-insecure behavior can turn into aggressive behavior over time. ◀

Given the high relevance of self-confidence for a healthy life, it is not surprising that
self-confidence trainings (also called social skills training, etc.) are standard in many

social, educational, and therapeutic institutions and are used in the latter for both prevention and therapy of various mental illnesses.

5.1.3 Why Train Self-Confidence with Dogs?

"Dogs have all the good qualities of humans, without simultaneously possessing their faults." (Quote attributed to Frederick the Great)

The idea of offering training with the support of therapy dogs arose during my professional activity as an animal-assisted therapist and my private cohabitation with dogs. The realization that dogs perceive human condition and behavior very accurately through their fine sensory channels and react to it was crucial for the development of the training. Studies of recent years confirm this or point to it (see Albuquerque et al., 2016; Müller et al., 2015).

But humans also have fine antennas for the insecurity or self-confidence of their counterpart. So what is the additional advantage of using dogs in a training for self-confidence? An interaction partner in the setting of a training acts as a mirror. It shows the practitioner through its reactions to him, how the participant affects him and how the participant behaves. And this brings us to the great advantage of practicing with a dog: Dogs do not have preconceived opinions, prejudices or the like based on appearances. They primarily react to the behavior of their counterpart. Therefore, in the analysis of their reaction to the participant, we have to subtract nothing or hardly anything, as we do, however, in the analysis of the behavior of a human interaction partner. In interpersonal interactions[3] the respective previous experiences and imprints play a role. This means that feedback is not exclusively based on the participant's specific behavior. Experiences and convictions of the feedback giver that are independent of this may also have influenced the feedback.

Example: Difference in reactions of humans and dogs to appearances

Participant 1 is severely overweight. A human counterpart may have prejudices about overweight (e.g., "those who are fat are lazy" or "those who are fat have little self-discipline"). Accordingly, these prejudices will influence the relationship and the behavioral dynamics between the participant and his interaction partner. The reactions of the counterpart to Participant 1 cannot be attributed solely to the participant's behavior, but are the result of a complex dynamic. The dog, on the other hand, primarily

---

[3] This is the case when they are not trained therapists, but when "laypeople" give each other feedback. For example, in the context of groups, where it is about building social skills and the group members give each other feedback.

reacts to the behavior of the person, regardless of whether the person is fat, has green hair, is dressed chic or sloppy, whether their teeth are crooked or straight.[4] ◄

Another advantage that speaks for the use of dogs is that they are much more authentic and direct in their reactions to their human counterparts than most other people.[5] The dog perceives something and reacts to it—without an intermediate filter of politeness, social desirability, or the like. Especially when self-confidence is practiced in groups and the group members engage in role-playing games that are subsequently analyzed, the feedback is often given very politely and hesitantly. The dog, on the other hand, shows his reaction to the behavior of his counterpart directly, unfiltered, and clearly, and that also *in* the situation. This also offers the opportunity to promote the feeling of self-efficacy in contact with the dog. The person does something and the dog reacts directly to it—this immediacy promotes the human sense of self-efficacy.

One could object that we live in a human world and that the potential participants in a self-confidence training have difficulties in self-confident behavior towards other people. So why practice with a dog despite all the advantages? Well, it actually makes no difference who the participant is dealing with. Because if you are insecure, you will also behave insecurely in contact with the dog. The insecurity may manifest itself differently or somewhat attenuated, but it is there, and we can work on it. It is always important to keep in mind: The training is about the participant's behavior, it is not about his counterpart! Developing self-confidence is about practicing and internalizing basic behaviors. Although my counterpart is present and reacts to me in his role as a mirror. But it is always exclusively about one's own behavior, one's own external effect, one's own relationship skills.

Summary: The Advantages of Using Dogs in the Context of Self-Confidence Training are:

- Fine perception of dogs regarding human condition and behavior
- Dogs' focus is on human behavior, not on appearances
- Dogs show authentic and clear reactions

---

[4] Of course, dogs also react to some extent to appearances, such as a walking aid or significant physical deviations from what they have learned as the norm. Here, experience plays a big role and thus the preparation of the dog. The more different people with different physical attributes a dog gets to know, the less he will react to external aspects in the future.

[5] However, this only applies to dogs that, like my therapy dogs, can live a balanced life with many freedoms and have undergone training in which they are not only allowed to maintain their natural and individual behaviors, but these are also actively promoted!

- Dogs react directly and immediately to the behavior of their counterpart, which favors the experience of self-efficacy

5.1.4   How Dogs React to Self-Confidence and Self-Insecurity

As previously stated, I assume that self-insecure and aggressive behavior are merely different expressions of the same inner state—namely self-insecurity. Since I do not allow people whose problem area includes open physically aggressive behavior to participate in animal-assisted therapy for the protection of my animals, I only distinguish between self-confident and self-insecure behavior towards the dog in dog-assisted self-confidence training. The latter can manifest itself in different ways: *shy* or *compensatory*. I speak of *shy* when the person behaves passively overall, shows little gesture and facial expression, tends to rigid behavior when carrying out something, rarely or only hesitantly shows feelings, and overall has a less present appearance. *Compensatory*, on the other hand, means that the person embarks on something like a "flight forward", i.e., feels insecure inside and tries to compensate for this feeling through dominant behavior, controlling behavior, or verbally aggressive behavior. Between the two variants of self-insecurity, there are various gradations and transitions. For practical work in the context of self-confidence training, only the basic differentiation between self-confident and self-insecure is relevant.

How exactly do dogs react to self-confidence and self-doubt? My observation is that they respond openly and relaxed when a person acts confidently towards them. Dogs react differently to self-insecure behavior. Uncertain behavior is harder for dogs to assess than clear, self-confident behavior. Thus, in my experience, dogs are themselves more uncertain when they work or interact with an uncertain person. To my knowledge, there are no studies yet that specifically investigate this correlation. However, there are various studies whose results suggest that dogs react to fearful behavior or hormonal stress factors in humans with stress and uncertain behavior (see Buttner et al., 2015; D'Aniello et al., 2018; O'Farrell, 1997; Schöberl et al., 2017; Sundman et al., 2019). Moreover, many training methods and dog training guides are now based on the realization that only a confident and therefore relaxed dog handler can be a good dog handler, as the confidence and thus relaxation of the human transfers to the dog (see Wischall-Wagner, 2019).

Now one must know the dog's temperament and previous experiences well in order to be able to read from its behavior whether it feels secure or insecure. I know my dogs very well—not least because I have trained them myself and have not only lived with them for many years, but work with them every day.

To illustrate how dogs can express security and insecurity in the same or different ways depending on their individual character, I describe in Table 5.1 the different behav-

Table 5.1   Reactions of the dog to confident and unconfident behavior

Situation	Reaction Giulio	Reaction Toni
When Giulio/Toni feels *confident* in dealing with the participant …	• He adjusts his pace to the participant • Shows spontaneous eye contact with the participant • Shows little interest in external distraction • *Actively seeks proximity to the participant* • Reacts joyfully to signals/commands of the participant	• He adjusts his pace to the participant • Shows spontaneous eye contact with the participant • Shows little interest in external distraction • *Maintains respectful distance from the participant* • Reacts joyfully to signals/commands of the participant
When Giulio/Toni feels *insecure* in dealing with the participant …	• *He walks and acts slower* • Shows less spontaneous eye contact with the participant • Sniffs more • *Keeps distance from the participant* • Reacts delayed or not at all to signals/commands of the participant	• *He walks and acts faster* • Shows less spontaneous eye contact with the participant • Sniffs more • *Is less distant towards the participant* • Reacts delayed or not at all to signals/commands of the participant

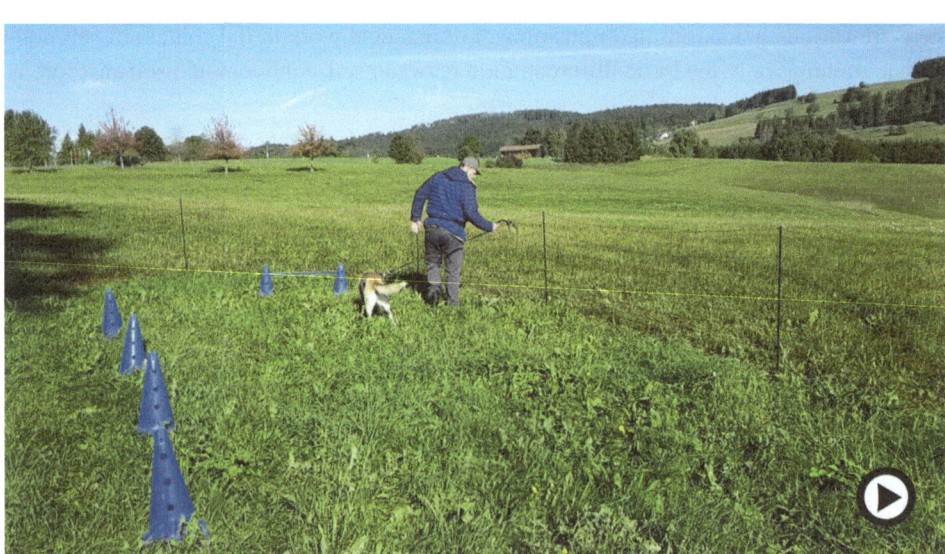

Here we can see that Giulio is sniffing quite a lot, walking with a rather large distance to the participant and that he is quite distracted. Now, Giulio gets simply pulled over, there is a lot of ambiguity, no direction is given and Giulio is distancing himself, sniffing, and just caring about other things. Giulio reacts slowly and resistant to the signals of the participant, to an extent that the participant almost isn´t able to get him moving. We can notice that both of them are acting past each other. Giulio is sniffing a lot to distract himself, is hesitant, and this is due to the fact that the leading by the participant is lacking of confidence and security.

Fig. 5.2   Giulio's reaction to insecure leadership (▶ https://doi.org/10.1007/000-axe)

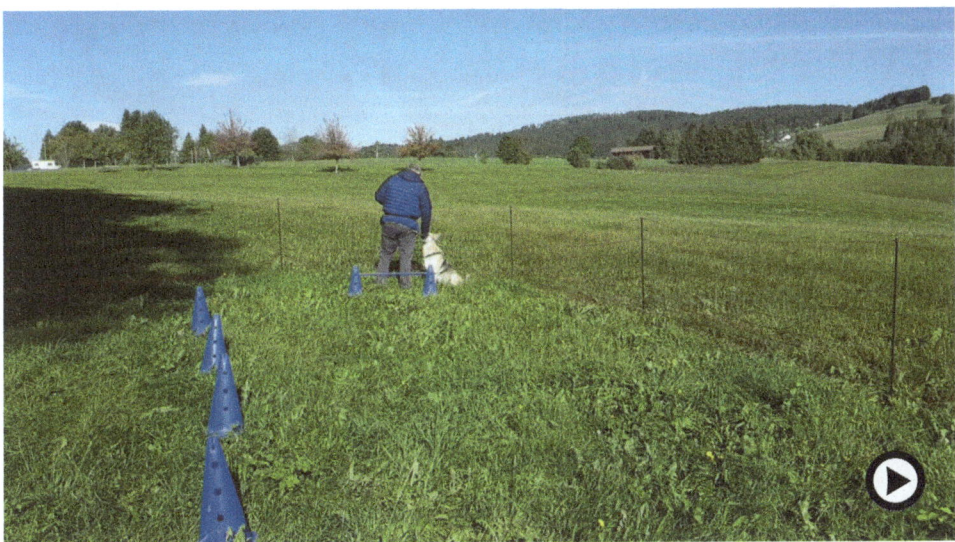

Here we can see the version of leading the dog where the participant has already some practice and is now able to lead in a more secure and confidant way. We can notice that by hearing that the participant talks to Giulio. We also see that Giulio is walking closer. Giulio is sniffing, but now we can see that the participant is conducting a little excercise to gain the attention back. We can see that there is more comunication, that Giulio is walking closer and is being more active. In summary we can see more comunication and an overall more secure leading of the dog.

Fig. 5.3   Giulio's reaction to secure leadership (▶ https://doi.org/10.1007/000-axc)

iors of Giulio (see for comparison Fig. 5.2 and 5.3) and Toni (see for comparison Fig. 5.4 and 5.5).

As can be seen from Table 5.1, it is worthwhile to pay attention to the speed of movement, the proximity-distance behavior, the reaction speed, and the spontaneous eye contact when assessing whether a dog is perceiving a sense of security or insecurity from a participant.

In general, it should be noted that some dogs are easier and others are somewhat harder to assess. Often, one has to look more attentive at the quieter dogs to correctly assess their condition.

Checklist: How to recognize if a dog feels secure or insecure when interacting with a participant?

To be able to recognize whether a dog feels secure or insecure when interacting with a participant, the following important points apply:

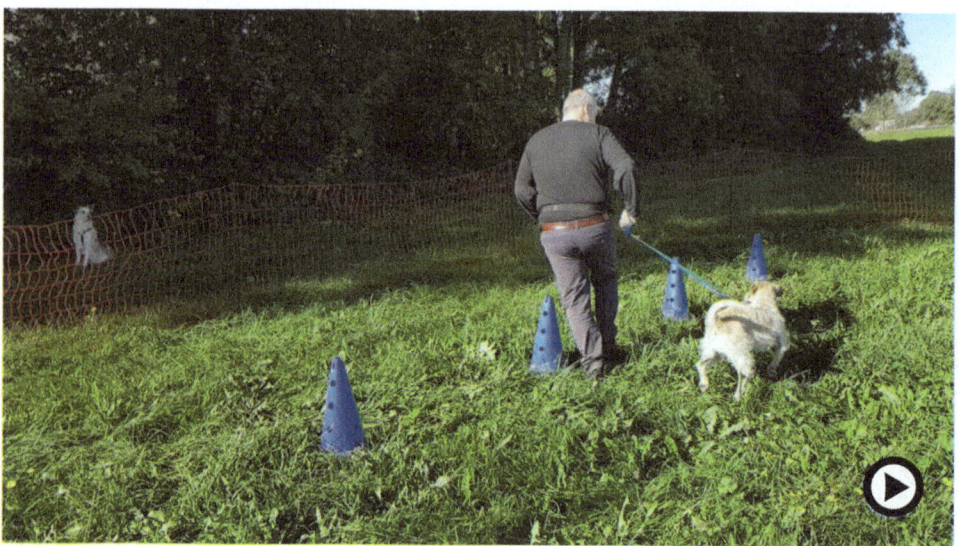

No comment because the video speaks for itself – we can observe an insecure leading of the dog

Fig. 5.4 Toni's reaction to insecure leadership (▶ https://doi.org/10.1007/000-axd)

- The therapist must…
  - know the dog well, have a close and good relationship with him, and have already experienced many different situations with him,
  - know how the dog behaves when he feels comfortable and secure,
  - know how the dog behaves when he feels insecure.
- The therapist is well advised in his assessment of the dog's behavior to pay particular attention to the following aspects:
  - The speed of movement
  - The proximity-distance behavior
  - The speed of reaction
  - The frequency of spontaneous eye contact

Hence, I can read from the reactions and general behavior of my dogs whether they feel secure or insecure when interacting with a participant. This in turn tells me whether the participant is acting securely or insecurely towards the dog. The behavior of my dogs shows me as a therapist whether the participant is self-confident or self-insecure and thus provides me with the basis for self-confidence training.

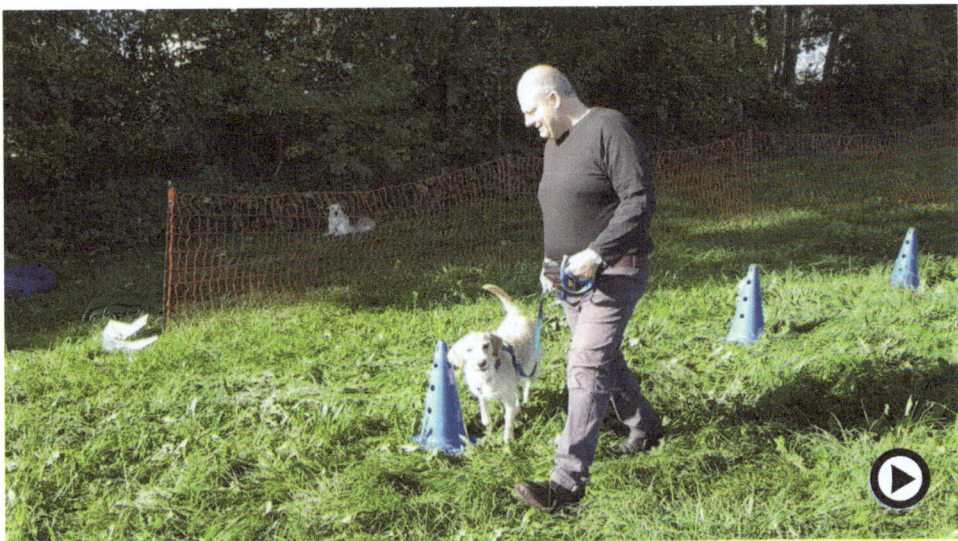

Here we can see a reduction of the use of the leash and in general more comunication between the participant and Toni. Toni, hence, slows down and is much more concentrated. The leading of the dog is getting more secure.

Fig. 5.5   Toni's reaction to secure leadership (▶ https://doi.org/10.1007/000-axb)

5.1.5   Self-Confident Behavior Towards a Dog

Having now explained what self-confidence is, why it is important, and how dogs react to self-confidence and self-insecurity, I would like to describe in this Sect. exactly what the self-confidence looks like that the participant learns in training with the dog.

Self-confidence towards a dog, as well as towards a human, manifests itself on various levels:

- On the one hand, through the behavior of a person that is immediately apparent, namely through voice and body language
- And on the other hand, through the not immediately apparent internal processes. These internal processes are thoughts, feelings, and attitudes. These largely determine a person's behavior as well as their general well-being.

The description of self-confident behavior in Table 5.2 with the addition of "adapted to the goal" may initially sound a bit cumbersome. However, it simply means the following: I must always have my specific goal in mind when dealing with the dog (for example: The dog should come to me on its own, or the dog should perform an exercise

Table 5.2 Manifestations of self-confidence towards a dog

	Levels of Mani-festation	Concrete Expression of Self-Assurance

Behavior	Voice	• Clear voice
		• Tone and volume are adapted to the respective goal, for example:
		   – Slightly deeper and quieter (Starting from the individual baseline, i.e., the individual way of speaking and expressing oneself), when the dog should show calm behavior
		   – Slightly brighter, louder and more motivating, when the dog should be active
		   – Warm and friendly when praising the dog

	Body Language	• Expressive body language
		• Muscle tone and movements are adapted to the respective goal, for example:
		   – More deliberate and slower (Again, starting from the individual baseline, i.e., the individual way of moving), when the dog should solve a task requiring concentration
		   – More dynamic and "sprightly", when the dog should do something active, for which he has to move quickly (jump)

Internal Processes	Thoughts and Feelings	• Constructive, strengthening thoughts
		• Feelings adapted to the goal, for example:
		   – Relaxation, when the dog should behave relaxed
		   – Joy when playing with the dog
		   – Concentration, when the dog should concentrate

	Attitude towards the Dog and Oneself	• Trust in the dog and appreciation for the dog • Self-worth and self-appreciation • IMPORTANT: The primary goal is never the task, but always the good relationship with the dog

calmly) and adjust my behavior accordingly. This means: If I want the dog to come to me motivated, then I will call him with a friendly and activating voice and display open body language. If I want the dog to relax, I will speak to him in a quiet, soothing voice and use calm gestures. The underlying eminently important thought to this is: If I want the dog to do or not do something specific, I must first consider what mental state the dog should be in to be able to perform this behavior, and then bring myself in this emotional state to convey it to the dog.

Example: What do I want from the dog and what must *I* as a human do for it

- *Initial situation:* I want the dog to walk calmly beside me.
- *Question:* How should the dog be internally prepared for this?
- *Answer:* The dog should be relaxed.
- *Question:* How can I put the dog in this state?

- *Answer:* By radiating calmness and thereby creating a relaxed working atmosphere.
- *Question:* How should I be internally prepared for this?
- *Answer:* I need to be relaxed and focus well on the dog and the situation.
- So, the circle is complete, and we can summarize: For the dog to walk calmly beside me, I must bring the dog into the necessary emotional state (namely relaxation) by being relaxed myself and thereby creating a relaxed atmosphere. ◄

▶   **Important!** For the dog to perform a behavior I desire, I must transfer the dog into the necessary emotional state by a) feeling this emotion myself and b) clearly conveying this emotion to the dog.

Beyond the immediate behavior, the participant's internal processes are a significant part of their self-confidence. A dog sees through "empty gestures". Therefore, the participant must work on their inner attitude beyond the level of behavior. The internal processes during or before an exercise with the dog are of great importance.

The participant may have fear-inducing thoughts beforehand ("Nothing will work, and I will embarrass myself"), which then lead to insecure-shy or insecure-compensating behavior towards the dog. This is the unfavorable case. Alternatively, the participant learns to have constructive thoughts and put themselves in a mood that is conducive to success. So instead of thinking "Nothing will work, and I will embarrass myself", they can practice thinking: "I will deal with the dog in a friendly and confident manner; then he will respond well to me, and we will master the exercise together". Such constructive thoughts can put the participant in a calm, optimistic mood, which then transfers to the dog through overall relaxed and open behavior.

The participant cannot expect the dog to perform a task with joy and concentration if the participant themselves does not enjoy the task and/or is unfocused. The dog, as mentioned, directly mirrors the participant. Therefore, when working with the dog, the participant must pay attention to their own emotional state and align it as much as possible with the dog's desired emotional state for the respective exercise.

Sometimes, particularly depressive participants argue at this point that they are in treatment for an affective disorder and cannot simply "feel joy". This is of course correct, however, participants suffering from depressive disorders *especially* benefit from this aspect of training with the dog! I have repeatedly seen individuals with diagnosed moderate depressive episodes blossom when they interact with the dog and motivate it. In these cases, it should be noted:

- It is normal for depressive participants to be initially skeptical and expect little change (this is part of the disorder)
- They need closer guidance than other participants
- And small successes must be celebrated greatly!

If he manages to find *a little* joy in a search game with the dog or to feel *a little* pride about a successful sit exercise, then this is a great progress for a depressed participant and should be named as such by the therapist.

Of course, the participant cannot "simply press a button" and be happy, but he can actively be present in the here and now with his thoughts and feelings, allow joy in dealing with the dog, and open himself up to good feelings. This is usually sufficient for mutual joy and fun to arise in playful exercises with the dog, and for the participant to interact exuberantly with the dog.

The attitude towards oneself and the dog, as well as behavior, thoughts, and feelings, is an important aspect of self-confidence. The attitude towards oneself and the dog not only decisively determines the participant's (spontaneous) behavior, which we try to balance in training through behavior modification and cognitive work. It's about something deeper. The attitude towards oneself reflects the basic attitude, the basic opinion about oneself with which the participant lives his life. The attitude towards the dog shows with which general attitude, with which expectation the participant encounters his environment and his fellow human beings. So it's about beliefs, about imprints.

In people with pronounced self-doubt, these beliefs are often dysfunctional, i.e., they harm the relationship with oneself and the relationship with others. Since these beliefs have usually been part of the participant's life for many years, it is not easy to shake them. Therefore, the therapist's claim for the training should always be based on a change in the here and now and in the specific situation with the dog. From the very beginning, the participant is taught the non-negotiable appreciation of the dog as an equal living being, thereby creating an atmosphere of mutual respect. He is encouraged to appreciate himself, his own developmental steps, and his own boundaries. For example, the participant's derogatory statements about himself are questioned and actively and repeatedly reformulated into appreciative sentences.

However, the development of self-confidence and trust in the dog also requires positive experiences—and that means: success experiences. Success in this case does not mean the dull, smooth execution of an exercise. Success means that the participant and the dog are increasingly growing together as a team. That both have fun with each other. That the participant feels: the dog sees me, reacts to me, enjoys working with me. The highest goal in every exercise, in every interaction with the dog, is therefore always the building and maintenance of the relationship. Through the good relationship with the dog, through the feeling of constant development of this relationship, the participant develops trust in the dog and trust in his own relationship skills.

Summary: Development of Self-Confidence

The development of self-confidence must be approached in a comprehensive manner. Concrete behaviors, expressed through body language and voice, are immediately apparent to the dog (and to people outside of training). Therefore, it is important to address this and help the participant express self-confidence through these channels. Body language and voice are the aspects that lie directly on the surface. They are influenced on the one hand by our conscious control, so that a certain active behavior change is possible. On the other hand, the inner processes and basic attitudes of the participant, which lie beneath the surface, determine how confidently he can interact with the dog (and outside of training with his fellow human beings). Therefore, in order for the learned self-confident behaviors not to remain abstract but to be filled with authenticity, it also requires change and development within the participant.

5.2 Content and Procedure of the Dog-Assisted Self-Confidence Training

The following provides an overview of the practical exercises used in self-confidence training as well as the specific procedure of the self-confidence training.

5.2.1 Overview: The Exercises Used in Training

In this section, I would like to explain which exercises I typically use during the self-confidence training. I do not follow a rigid plan, but rather adapt the exercises to the individual competencies and, above all, to the focus determined together with the participant at the beginning.

For example, if a participant already has good skills in dealing with others but lacks self-confidence, I will focus on leash-free exercises quite early on. This is because a participant with such a focus should be able to experience early in the training that they do not need a leash to interact with the dog. They should experience that they can trust themselves and their skills in dealing with the dog. If a participant, on the other hand, has little sense of themselves and their counterpart, I will focus with them on simple exercises such as right and left turns on the leash. In this way, they can develop more mindfulness for themselves and their impact, as well as for the dog and its reactions. In this exercise, they learn to coordinate their body language and voice according to their goal. Moreover, the exercise only works if they put themselves in the dog's perspective and send signals to the dog that are understandable for it.

This means that I set up an individual training plan with exercises that match their focus for each participant. In Table 5.3, I provide an overview of the exercises I use most frequently in the training. All the exercises listed there serve to increase self-confidence. Therefore, in *every* one of these exercises, confident body language, a confident voice, confident internal processes, and a confident attitude are practiced and learned (see Table 5.2). Thus, the training involves approaching each exercise with an open body language adapted to the goal, a clear voice adapted to the goal, as well as with constructive thoughts and feelings, and a fundamentally appreciative and trusting attitude towards

Table 5.3 Exercises within the framework of self-confidence training

With or without leash	Exercise	What does the participant need to do specifically?	What does the participant learn from this exercise?
Possible both with and without leash	Leading the dog on a straight path	• Have a clear path in mind • Motivate the dog to walk along (dog should not stop) • Limit the dog (dog should not run ahead)	• Confident walking and acting • Motivating their counterpart • Limiting their counterpart
Possible with or without a leash	Right and left turns with the dog	• Have a clear path in mind • Motivate the dog to walk along (the dog should not stop) • Limit the dog (the dog should not run ahead) • Recognize which signals the dog needs to know which direction to go • Send clear signals to the dog	• Confident walking and acting • Motivating your counterpart • Limiting your counterpart • Perspective taking, empathy • Clarity • Interplay of body language and voice
Possible with or without a leash	Slalom	• Have a clear path in mind • Motivate the dog to run along (the dog should not stop) • Limit the dog (the dog should not run ahead) • Recognize which signals the dog needs to correctly run around the pylons • Send clear signals to the dog	• Confident walking and acting • Motivating your counterpart • Limiting your counterpart • Perspective taking, empathy • Interplay of body language and voice • Clarity
Possible with or without a leash	Obstacle (see Fig. 5.6)	• Focus on the obstacle • Recognize which signals the dog needs to jump over the obstacle • Get the dog to jump through dynamic body language and voice • Send clear signals to the dog	• Confident walking and acting • Perspective taking, empathy • Motivating your counterpart • Interplay of body language and voice • Clarity

(continued)

Table 5.3 (continued)

With or without leash	Exercise	What does the participant need to do specifically?	What does the participant learn from this exercise?
Possible with or without a leash	Course (i.e., combination of individual exercises, for example, slalom and obstacle)	• Depends on the individual exercises that build up the course • In addition: Transitions between exercises must be clearly indicated; concentration must be maintained	• Depends on the individual exercises that build up the course • In addition: – Concentration – Readiness to act – Flexibility
Possible with or without a leash	Commands via visual and auditory signals • *Sit* • *Down* • *Wait* • *Come*	• Know what I want • Meaningful timing • Send clear signals to the dog	• Clarity • Determination • Interplay of body language and voice
Exclusively without a leash	Call the dog from a distance (see Fig. 5.7)	• Be convinced that the dog will come • Friendly, motivating call with open body language • Send clear signals to the dog	• Positive, open attitude towards myself and the dog • Confident action • Motivate the counterpart • Clarity
Exclusively without a leash	Let the dog search for something	• Concentration on the object to be searched • Recognize which signals the dog needs to know that (and possibly where) he should search • Clear, motivating guidance of the dog to search	• Concentration • Perspective taking, empathy • Trust (in own competencies for guidance and in the dog's search skills) • Motivate the counterpart • Clarity

oneself and the dog. This is the common denominator of all exercises. In addition, a specific aspect of self-confidence can be particularly practiced in each individual exercise. These additional points are listed in the last column of Table 5.3.

The points listed in the last column of Table 5.3 indicate how the participant can work on different aspects of their own self-confidence by training with the dog. When we work on an exercise with the dog—for example, on the obstacle (see Fig. 5.6) or on calling from a distance (see Fig. 5.7)—I point out before, during, and after the exercise the aspects of self-confidence that the participant is currently training.

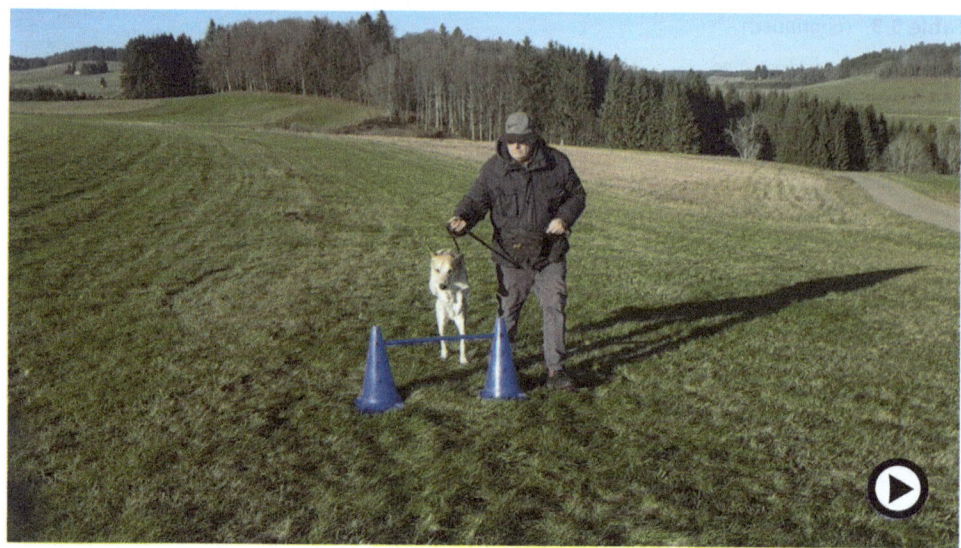

Participant: „Fine! Fine! Sit"

Fig. 5.6 Obstacle (▶ https://doi.org/10.1007/000-axf)

In all the exercises that the participant carries out as part of the self-confidence training, I always make sure to repeatedly relate to the everyday and relationship difficulties
rooted in the participant's previous self-insecurity. This transfer is of high importance for
the medium and long-term effects of the self-confidence training. Only in this way can
the successes from working with the dog be transferred to the participant's life. More on
this later. First, I will present the process of the initial consultation and the further course
of the training.

5.2.2 Course of the Training

5.2.2.1 The Initial Consultation—Introduction to the Training

The initial consultation shapes the further course of the animal-assisted therapy and
includes mutual acquaintance, clarification of conditions, introduction to the self-confidence training, and determination of the goal and focus of the further sessions.

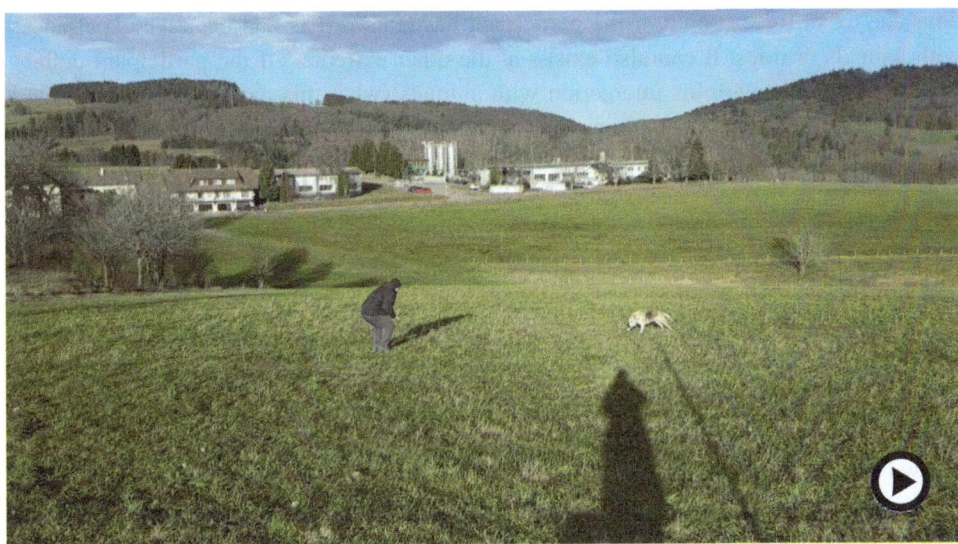

Participant: „Giulio! Giulio!"

Fig. 5.7 Calling the dog from a distance (▶ https://doi.org/10.1007/000-axg)

5.2.2.1.1 Setting of the Initial Consultation

The initial consultation takes place in a quiet room where an undisturbed and open conversation can be held and where the dogs are familiar and comfortable. Usually, only one dog is present, namely the one with whom I will probably work with the participant in the future.[6] The participant first gets to know the dog, with the first encounter usually taking place in such a way that the participant enters the room, we greet each other, and the dog comes to the participant, sniffs, and allows itself to be petted and greeted. Afterward, the dog either lies down on its resting place or joins the seating group, where I sit with the participant and conduct the initial consultation.

5.2.2.1.2 Clarification of Important Questions and Framework Conditions

At the beginning, the participant can ask his questions if he has any right from the start. Otherwise, I start asking, first about his relationship with dogs and animals in general. This question is important to get to know the participant and to assess whether the participant starts the therapy without prejudice or not. Prejudice regarding working with

---

[6]Sometimes it may happen that I foresee one of the dogs as a training partner and then realize during the initial consultation that one of the other two dogs would be better suited for working on the topic or the respective participant. Then a change takes place. Also, during the course of the training, I occasionally switch the dogs depending on the course and focus.

dogs can exist, for example, if the participant has fears or has had negative experiences with animals or dogs. It can also exist—at the other extreme—if the participant defines his self-esteem through his interaction with animals (what this may mean for therapy, I explain in Sect. 5.3.1). Depending on this, it may then be necessary to precede certain steps before starting the self-confidence training, such as reducing fears or clarifying discussions on certain aspects.

In the next step, I explain the framework conditions of animal-assisted therapy, such as the duration of the sessions, the future meeting point, and other practical aspects. I also now explain the rules of behavior towards the dog and discuss these in depth with the participant if necessary. As already explained elsewhere, these rules are as follows:

- **Respect for the dog**: We meet the dog at eye-to-eye level and respect his boundaries
- **Perception of the dog as an individual**: We perceive the dog as an individual with its own needs, its own character, and its own will, and treat it accordingly
- **Working with the dog means working on ourselves**: We use the exchange with the dog to learn something about ourselves. Through his behavior, the dog continuously and unadulteratedly gives us feedback on how we affect him. In our relationship with the dog, we have the opportunity to reflect on ourselves and change our behavior.

5.2.2.1.3 Assessment of the Participant's Self-Confidence

To determine the goal and focus, it is first necessary to assess how self-confident or self*un*confident the participant is at the present time. For this, I discuss the participant's view of himself:

- How self-confident does he generally consider himself to be?
- In which situations does he feel self-confident?
- In which situations does he feel self-insecure?
- What understanding of self-confidence and self-insecurity does he have?

People who tend to compensate for their insecurity (see Sect. 5.1.2), in my experience, often tend to confuse self-confident behavior with aggressive behavior. When I ask how they think self-confident behavior manifests itself, attributes such as "loud voice", "dominant appearance" or "being able to assert oneself" are often mentioned. The fact that willingness to compromise, flexibility, and friendliness are central aspects of self-confident behavior is surprising and often questioned ("but then the other person will walk all over me"). So, at the beginning, a deeper discussion or psychoeducation may be necessary to start from a common denominator.

▶   **Important!** Before starting the training, it should be ensured that the therapist and participant have the same understanding of self-confidence and are thus working towards the same goal!

5.2.2.1.4 Setting Therapy Goals and Focus

If it turns out in the conversation that the participant has been suffering from self-doubt either since forever or due to a life-changing event or an acute crisis, the specific goal is now defined. It can be quite global: *Increasing general self-confidence* or *Developing more self-esteem.* However, the more individual and specific the participant's goal can be formulated, the more targeted and better the therapy can be designed. It can also be better checked whether something changes during the process of therapy. It is therefore worth probing a little more at the beginning and hence formulate a tangible goal together with the participant. Concrete examples of such goals are: *Develop more self-confidence when I dare to try something new* or *Dare to approach new people* or *Reduce my fear of embarrassing myself* or *Worry less about the opinions of others.*

In the next step, it is then discussed how exactly the dog can be used to work towards this goal. I first explain to the participant why and how self-confidence can be practiced with the dog. At the same time, correspondences of the aspects of self-confidence practiced in dealing with the dog are sought in the participant's everyday life. For example, building and maintaining eye contact with the dog, praising and friendly addressing are important aspects of self-confident interaction with a dog. In interpersonal relationships, praising corresponds to the expression of appreciation or affection. And the competence to be able to show appreciation and affection adequately is also an important part of self-confidence. If someone has previously struggled with this in the interpersonal area, then I will practice the appropriate praising of the dog more intensively in the upcoming sessions and in the subsequent conversations, the participant and I reflect on what learning experiences he is making and which aspects can be transferred to his everyday life.

5.2.2.1.5 Explaining that Self-Confidence Can Be Well Trained with Dogs

The initial consultation also serves to convey to the participant why he can improve his self-confidence in training with the dog. Because the participant may rightly question why a dog is used at this point and why he is instead working with a human counterpart. For this, I explain the reasons mentioned in Sects. 5.1.3 and 5.1.4 with a special focus on the fact that dogs react to human self-confidence with self-confident behavior and to human insecurity with self-uncertain behavior. The participant is taught that he gets feedback on his own appearance and effect through the behavior of the dog. Through this feedback, he has the opportunity to work on his behavior and inner state and gradually build up more self-confidence.

▶   **Important!** The reactions of a dog to human behavior are to be understood as a mirror and allow the human to consciously understand his own behavior, reflect on it and (in the last and most important step) gradually change towards more self-confidence.

5.2.2.1.6 Joint Development of Self-Confident Behavior Towards a Dog

Together with the participant, I then define the exact aspects of self-confident behavior towards a dog in the last part of the initial conversation (see Table 5.2). At this point, it is determined which exact behaviors with the dog will be practiced in further training. It is important to constantly seek the connection and correspondences in his real interpersonal relationships with the participant.

In the discussion of behavior and internal processes in self-confidence (see Table 5.2), I devote time and attention to each individual aspect. I make sure to express the individual points in the participant's language, so as not to lose him because of terminology that appears artificial to him. Together with the participant, I also highlight which aspects of self-confidence have been most difficult for him so far and have a connection to his therapy goal. These points will then be the focus of the training. Sometimes this changes over time, or the participant only realizes in practice what is really difficult for him, and this changes the goal and focus.

▶   **Important!** The terminology used should correspond to the participant's normal language use. As a therapist, I don't "break a sweat" if I adopt some of the participant's colloquial expressions for better understanding.

Summary: Procedure and Contents of the Initial Conversation

- Mutual introduction, including getting to know the therapy dog
- Clarifying to what extent there is impartiality regarding animal-assisted therapy (otherwise, other sessions may be necessary before self-assurance training)
- Demonstration of the possibilities of animal-assisted therapy
    - Depending on the participant's specific topic
    - Always important: explain why self-confidence can be practiced with the dog (see Sect. 5.1.3)
- Explanation of the therapy framework conditions
    - Practical aspects such as duration of sessions and answering possbible
    - Introducing the rules of behavior towards the dogs (see Sect. 3.4.2)
- Discussion of the participant's self-confidence
    - Specific questions to classify the participant's view of himself
    - Ensure the same understanding of the term "self-confidence"
- Explanation of what self-confidence towards a dog looks like in concrete terms (see Table 5.2)
- Determination of the goal and focus of animal-assisted therapy

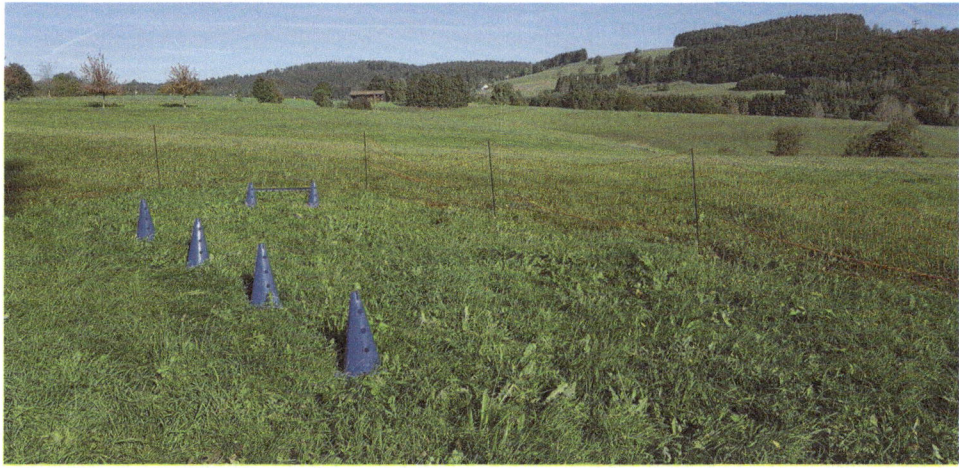

Fig. 5.8 Exercise area

5.2.2.2 Course of Training: Working on Change

After the foundation for the self-confidence training was laid in the initial conversation (see Sect. 5.2.2.1), we move on to the practical sessions in the following meetings. This involves doing simple exercises with the dog—always with the aim of gradually increasing the participant's self-confidence. The focus, as already mentioned, is not on the smooth execution of the exercise, but on how the participant feels during the process, how they behave towards the dog, and how they internally process the course of the exercise.

▶   **Important!** The focus during the practical exercises with the dog is on how the participant feels during the execution of the exercises, how they behave towards the dog, and how they internally process the course and outcome of the exercise.

So we start the training. First, it is now about the participant and the dog getting into contact with each other and starting to engage with each other. Practically, this means that I go with the participant and the dog to a quiet exercise area (see fig. 5.8). There, the participant walks the first round over the exercise area with the dog on a leash. This first joint walk is important to me because it gives me the opportunity to recognize what practical skills the participant already has. In the preliminary discussions, the participant reports on their general self-confidence and whether they have previous experience with dogs or not. However, we can only recognize how self-confident (or not) the participant actually is when actually dealing with the dog.

Example: First practical session

Participant 2 suffers from depressive symptoms and comes to animal-assisted therapy due to a significantly reduced sense of self-worth and self-doubt in social situations. She has her first practical session with the experienced therapy dog Giulio. She is friendly and open towards Giulio and towards me as a therapist. When she is supposed to walk a bit with Giulio on a leash, she keeps turning to me and reassures herself whether she is doing everything right. Giulio senses her fearful attitude, her lack of concentration on him, which leads to Giulio withdrawing his attention from her, sniffing, doing "his thing". Participant 2 notices that Giulio stops a lot and sniffs. Half-heartedly, she tries to motivate him to continue walking. A questioning, quiet "Come …" while she herself hesitates from one foot to the other, wants to start walking, but doesn't dare because she fears Giulio will not follow her—which is exactly what happens due to the uncertain address and passive body language. Participant 2 then reacts to Giulio's undeterred sniffing with insecure laughter and jokes, with the latter devaluing herself and reinforcing her insecurity ("even Giulio doesn't take me seriously"). ◄

During the first practical session, I observe how the participant spontaneously, i.e. without specific instructions or hints from me, interacts with the dog.

- Do they talk to the dog on their own?
- Do they praise the dog?
- Do they expect attention from the dog?
- Do they use the leash as a means of pressure?
- Are they passive?
- What do facial expressions and body language reveal?
- What does the participant spontaneously express during the interaction with the dog?

These are just some examples of aspects that I pay attention to when the participant interacts with the dog. It's about paying attention to details and at the same time developing a holistic idea of which beliefs and fears become active in the participant during interaction with the dog. Every person reacts differently when given a task. In our context, the task is to lead the dog. Depending on prior experiences, personality, and degree of self-confidence, a person handles this task differently.

My observations regarding the different handling of this task can be summarized as follows (simplified): The more self-confident a person is, the more open, relaxed, and spontaneous they interact with the dog. The less self-confident a person is, the more the topic of *control* comes into play. Because insecurity is linked to fear, and fear leads to attempts to control. This striving for control can manifest in different ways. It may be that the participant tries to control their own behavior as much as possible to avoid making mistakes. It could also be that they strive to control the dog's behavior by interacting with the dog through pressure and restriction. Or the issue of control manifests itself primarily within the participant—as fear of losing control, for example. Or as an expectation of the dog, namely, that it behaves very controlled, i.e., does not show spontaneous behaviors.

> ▶   **Important!** The more self-confident a person is, the more open, relaxed, and spontaneous they interact with the dog. The less self- confident a person is, the more controlled their behavior is and the more they try to control the dog, or they fear losing control or expect controlled behavior from the dog.

So, in the first training session, I get a concrete picture of the participant's level of self-confidence. This is openly discussed with the participant in the discussion that follows the practical part of the session, and based on this conversation, the focus of the further sessions is determined.

Example: Debriefing following the first practical session

Let's go back to the example of participant 2: After the session, I discuss with her the reasons why Giulio did not respond to her. For her, only the feeling of failure and defeat remains. Therefore, it is essential to analyze the situation together. We discuss that her inner insecurity (i.e., her self-doubt, her fear of failure, her fear of losing control) is expressed in a lack of concentration on Giulio, a soft voice, a questioning tone, and unclear, passive body language. Internally, she already assumes that Giulio will not follow her, which in turn scares her, and which fulfills itself in the sense of a self-fulfilling prophecy. Because her insecure behavior leads to Giulio turning away from her internally and making decisions himself. We record this dynamic on a flipchart, which allows participant 2 to understand the causal relationships. After that, we think together about how she can break out of this cycle and become more self-confident. ◀

In almost every participant, the analysis of the first session shows that it is necessary to approach from several sides in order to help the participant gain more self-confidence (see Table 5.4).

For some participants, cognitive work is more important than behavior changes. For others, behavior change is paramount. For yet others, experiencing success is most important. However, all three points are usually to be considered for each participant, so that the participant can gradually approach his goal of higher self-confidence in the following sessions.

Excursion: Humility

Humility has a sometimes a somewhat negative connotation. Therefore, I will explain here in more detail how I understand this term.

Table 5.4 Levels of action for building self-confidence

Levels of action	Explanation	Specific for participant 2
Cognitive work	Replacing obstructive thoughts with supportive, strengthening thoughts	Moving from "I will embarrass myself" to "I can do this!" Moving from "The dog doesn't take me seriously" to "I will act confidently, and then the dog will respond well to me"
Behavior change	Replacing insecure behavior with confident behavior	Moving from insecure behavior to: Focusing on the dog Upright posture Firm, clear voice Saying "Come" and starting to walk with the conviction that the dog will follow
Enabling success experiences	Concerns the therapist: exercises with a high probability of success for the participant are selected, successes are highlighted	Simple exercises are selected for participant 2 Successes are emphasized during the exercises, repeated at the end of the session Overall, joy about a successful exercise is openly and intensely shown to further motivate the participant
In the later course: development of a *healthy humility*.	Develop self-confidence through successes, without overestimating oneself or resting on one's laurels. Each session with the dog represents a new challenge; the development process is never completed	See example for participant 2 in the further course

By *healthy humility* (see Table 5.4), the following is meant: The participant (or more generally the dog handler) is always aware that the successful completion of an exercise is no guarantee for the future. The human must remain alert, attentive, and focused when interacting with the dog, only then can the dog and human bring out their best in an exercise or situation. The dog notices when the human is unfocused due to overconfidence or is half-hearted about his task. Healthy humility is one of the keys to long-term success in working with the dog.

Especially when self-confidence training is used to improve the participant's professional leadership skills, the aspect of healthy humility is essential. Other leadership trainings in this area are based on leadership concepts that understand humility as the highest possible level of leadership behavior (Collins, 2001).

Now, various practical exercises with the dog are used, which build on each other and become increasingly demanding and complex over time. In the first session, as described above, the participant initially leads the dog intuitively on a leash. In the following sessions, the leash handling spontaneously shown by the participant is gradually improved and practiced in increasingly difficult situations. For this, he is accompanied by me at his own pace and receives the necessary assistance, instructions, and feedback so that he can lead the dog with increasing confidence.

> **Example: Second Practical Session**
>
> In the second practical session with participant 2, the aim is now to start with cognitive work and behavior change. I discuss with her again the constructive thoughts formulated last time, "I can do this!" and "I will act confidently and then Giulio will react well to me". We then go together to the training area and briefly discuss what we are going to do today. Participant 2 is to practice leading Giulio confidently on different routes (in a circle, straight ahead, with turns to the left and right, at different walking speeds). The first exercise is leading Giulio along the boundary of the training area. The leash should be loose, Giulio should walk next to participant 2, and the two should not stop. Before starting this exercise, I repeat the constructive thoughts with participant 2. I will do this in the first sessions before each exercise until participant 2 has sufficiently internalized these thoughts. At the same time, I give her practical tips on how she can lead Giulio more confidently along the fence (= work on behavior). I encourage her to focus exclusively on Giulio and herself, to walk upright and maintain an action-ready, active body tension. If Giulio, for example, shows signs of wanting to stop, participant 2 should react immediately, i.e., continue walking and speak to him in a friendly and encouraging manner ("Come on, let's go!"). She can implement everything very well and successfully completes the exercise. I am happy with her, underline her performance, draw a comparison to the last time and emphasize what she did well today and differently from the last time. ◄

The successes are "enjoyed" with the participant and, depending on the participant's wish, also recorded in writing. The beneficial processing and recording of successful experiences are at least as important as the actual practice, as they serve to promote self-confidence and the feeling of self-efficacy. These are then essential prerequisites for daring to take the step into more difficult exercises, and for being able to generalize from working with the dog to other areas of life. In the course of therapy, I like to draw comparisons with the difficulties at the beginning of therapy: "Do you remember how at the beginning you didn't even know how to hold the leash in your hand? Or how you couldn't encourage Giulio to keep walking? And now? Now you perform the exercises like a pro! If you embrace a challenge, if you appear confident both internally and externally, you can achieve more than you can imagine!"

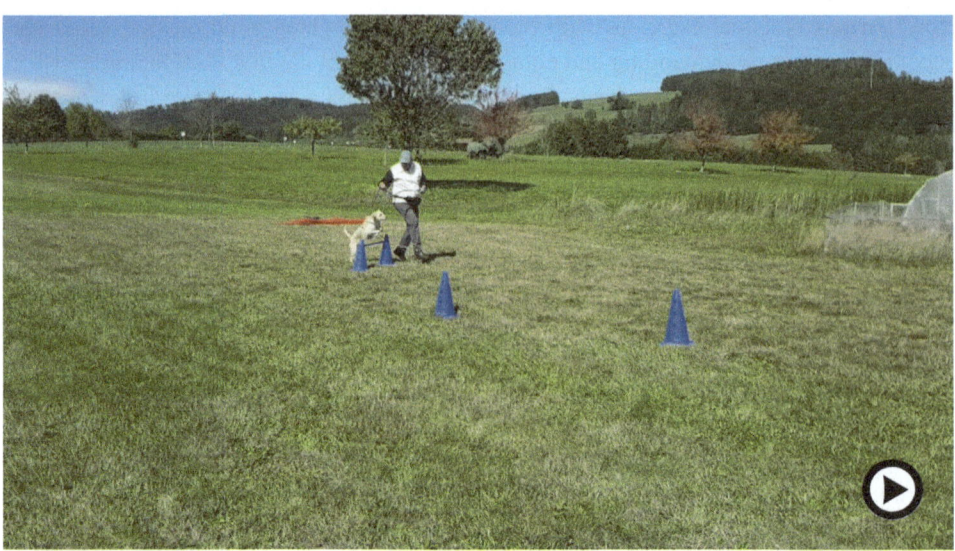

Here we see the conduction of a course, which consists of walking Toni through a slalom and than making him jump an obstacle. We can see a very nice interaction between the participant and Toni. The participant establishes a positive contact with Toni and maintains eyecontact with him. The result is that they are collaborating as a team, and getting to this point is what we consider a secure and confident leading of the dog.

Fig. 5.9 Obstacle Course (▶ https://doi.org/10.1007/000-axh)

5.2.2.2.1 Obstacle Course Work

In almost all self-confidence trainings, I like to use obstacle courses (usually towards the end of the training). Because—as can be seen in Table 5.3—the participant can learn various things during the obstacle course work. The dog must be clearly guided in an obstacle course so that it can go through the different stations of the course successfully with the participant (see Fig. 5.9). Each station, each building block of a course, also offers different exercise opportunities.

It is important to clearly distinguish the obstacle course work taking place in the context of self-confidence training from the well-known agility training[7] . The equipment used is the same, the sequence of exercises is similar. However, the focus is completely different. Agility training is about the dog showing good performance.[8] In my self-con-

---

[7] Also from dog sports or related methods and exercises from dog training.

[8] Of course, human support and a harmonious human-dog relationship are also needed in agility or dog sports for a good performance of the dog. However, the focus is primarily on the performance of the dog.

fidence training, it's about the participant. The participant should guide the dog clearly, confidently, and sovereignly so that it has no choice but to get through the course well. Or to put it another way: the participant should lead the dog so confidently that even an untrained dog would successfully get through the course. It's all about the appearance, the inner attitude, and the general effect of the participant.

▶   **Important!** The obstacle course work in the context of self-confidence train-
    ing focuses on the behavior of the participant and not the performance of the
    dog. So it should not be confused with agility training.

As mentioned, obstacle course work with the dog offers several opportunities to promote the participant's self-confidence. I usually compose the course from three components: a slalom course, one or more obstacles, and one or more sit or down exercises. In prin-ciple, the course can be modified or expanded with other exercises as desired. However, for me, the mentioned exercises have crystallized as ideal components for training self-confidence. The change from the slalom directly into the obstacle exercise requires the quick and clear activation of the dog. When changing from the obstacle directly into the subsequent sit or down exercise, the participant must slow down the dog and bring it into the necessary relaxation. In the sequence of the three components, it is trained to concen-trate, to be ready to act, and to adapt one's own behavior flexibly to one's own goals.

5.2.2.2.2 Exercises Without a Leash

As can be seen in Table 5.3, most exercises (i.e., all exercises except *calling the dog from a distance* and *letting the dog search for something*) can be performed both with and without a leash. The start of working without a leash often represents an important step. The greatest challenge for the participant is on the mental level. Even though the partici-pant learns from the beginning to always keep the leash loose, so the leash hardly has a function, it still provides the participant with a certain external security. The leash feels like a safety net. And this external security is now taken away from him. Now it becomes clear at which development point in terms of self-confidence a participant is.

Example: Exercises without a leash

Participant 2 works without a leash with Giulio for the first time. We introduce this playfully by initiating a search game. Participant 2 implements the instructions well: she motivates Giulio for playful interaction through an inviting, activating voice and dynamic body language. Then we move on to leading Giulio without a leash. The goal here is to lead Giulio just as she has done on the leash so far. In the first run (she is supposed to walk a straight path with Giulio), Participant 2 changes her behavior. It is noticeable that she is insecure due to the absence of the leash. She keeps turning to Giulio, bends slightly down to him, says "Come" too often and with a fearful-ques-tioning undertone. Giulio walks next to her, but at a much greater distance than usual.

The pressure from the constant repetition of the command makes him seek distance. At the end of the run, the participant is visibly stressed; the free leading of Giulio was a real struggle for her due to her constant striving for control and monitoring of Giulio. We do a relaxation exercise to help her letting go of fear. We then formulate helpful sentences,[9] that help her to regain confident leadership of Giulio despite the missing leash. "Less is more!" (regarding addressing Giulio) and "Giulio will follow me if I speak to him in a friendly-motivating manner when I start walking and then calmly and decisively go my way" help her. Participant 2 manages the implementation. We initially choose only short and simple routes, so Participant 2 can gain self-confidence from her successes and become increasingly confident. ◄

The example of Participant 2 shows that some participants initially tend to do too much when working without a leash. They start acting, become restless and strive for control of the dog, instead of implementing the learned self-confident behaviors. This is the case when self-confidence is still unstable, when the participant quickly falls back into his self-insecure behavior pattern. Sometimes it can also happen that the participant is at the point where he takes success for granted, lacking the necessary healthy humility (see Table 5.4). Then it can happen that the participant does too little to guide and lead the dog without a leash. The result is then similar, namely that the dog keeps a distance, or pursues his own goals, because he lacks guidance. The goal in both cases is to bring the participant to lead the dog as confidently and self-assuredly as he has previously done with the help of the leash.

5.2.2.3 Transfer of Learned Skills to Everyday Life

As already mentioned, the transfer of what has been learned into the participant's everyday life is crucial for whether he can benefit from the self-confidence training in the medium and long term (Mörtl et al., 2008). What points should be considered so that the participant can transfer the self-confidence from the training into his everyday life and thus become more self-confident in his life and his relationships?

In my experience, the transfer of what has been learned into everyday life is most successful when the participant independently reflects on it. Such reflections can best be promoted by me, as a therapist, asking questions.

Example: Transfer of Learned Skills to Everyday Life

Participant 3 often feels lonely in everyday life. She would like to have deeper relationships with people and make friends, but so far she has not been successful. Over time, she has developed the opinion that she is not lovable. In the fourth session of the self-confidence training with Cleo, Participant 3 begins to work without a leash for

---

[9] See "Cognitive Work" in Table 5.4.

the first time. She is supposed to get Cleo to follow her voluntarily across the training ground without any commands. Participant 3 can't think of a strategy to get Cleo to follow voluntarily.

Here, in the sense of the action levels for the development of self-confidence described in Table 5.4, a multi-layered approach is necessary. In the first step, I turn to cognitive work with Participant 3. She implicitly assumes that Cleo will only follow her if she gives her the command to do so. The idea that Cleo would follow her voluntarily is still foreign to Participant 3. With the help of appropriate questions, Participant 3 and I verbalize her implicit, obstructive thought "Cleo only comes when I command her to do so". From this thought, we come to the underlying belief "I am not lovable". Now we formulate a cognitive counter-model together. For the training, we use the sentence "I am lovable and Cleo likes to follow me." Another obstructive thought of Participant 3 emerges, namely: "The exercise must succeed, otherwise I will embarrass myself." This thought builds pressure, and she passes this pressure on to Cleo through an overall restrictive and demanding behavior, to which Cleo reacts with distance. So we also formulate a constructive counter-thought to this, namely: "I invite Cleo to follow me. But she can also choose not to follow me." In the second step, we turn to the necessary behavior change. I guide Participant 3 on how to build a loving, non-demanding contact with Cleo through her voice and body language. The beneficial thoughts are repeated out loud again before the exercise. Then it can start. As previously discussed, she bends down to Cleo, strokes her and speaks to her in a soft voice. Then she stands up and walks away relaxed and determined. Cleo follows her.

Following the session, I now turn to the transfer of today's experience to Participant 3's everyday life. Through various questions, such as "Do you know the feeling you had at the beginning of the session when you didn't know how to get Cleo to follow you, from other situations?" or "Can you transfer anything from what you learned today in contact with Cleo to other relationships?", she comes to an important conclusion. As before with Cleo, she tries in everyday life to force friendship and close contact by building pressure and reacting hurt to lack of closeness. The other person then usually keeps their distance. Her take-home message today is that in the future she wants to adopt a non-demanding, but friendly and open attitude in contact with others. We formulate helpful thoughts for this, which Participant 3 writes down and wants to try out in everyday life. ◄

As this example shows, it is important during the course of the self-confidence training to always bear in mind the specific difficulties and insecurities the participant experiences in everyday life. Does he feel misunderstood in his relationships? Does he have a issues with his boss? Does he not dare to express his opinion? Is there frequent conflict in the partnership? Only if the therapist, constantly bears these problems in mind, can he obtain results from the work with the dog. Only then can he help the participant to transfer the established self-confidence to his relationships and everyday life.

▶   **Important!** Only the transfer of what has been learned to everyday life and relationships allows the participant to benefit from the self-confidence training in the long term.

5.2.2.4 Failure as the Key to Success

In self-confidence training, successes are important because they allow the participant to see progress and hence to remain motivated. However, the failed exercises with the dog, the so-called failures, are much more significant and progressive. They point out aspects of self-confidence that the participant cannot yet implement, and they offer him the opportunity to learn how to deal with setbacks constructively—a central aspect especially for depressive participants.

Example: Failure as the Key to Success

Back to participant 2. In the previous exercises, participant 2 was able to orient herself by the fence as a boundary. In the current exercise, we take a step further and detach ourselves from the fence. Participant 2 is now supposed to lead Giulio on a route over the training ground that she invents herself. She chooses a triangle. The new challenge is that the route only exists in her head, she has no external help by the limitations of the fence, and the route includes one or more changes of direction. So it requires special concentration and clear communication with Giulio. We discuss how she can clearly indicate a change of direction to Giulio: if she turns in the direction in which Giulio is already walking, she must limit him using her body language. If, on the other hand, she turns in the opposite direction, she must motivate Giulio to follow her. Participant 2 starts the exercise and only manages the route with difficulty. She finds it hard to clearly indicate the direction to Giulio. She hesitates, briefly indicates movements, then discards them again. Giulio is thereby irritated and is forced by the lack of guidance from participant 2 to make his own decisions. The result is that the triangle becomes an egg, which is awkwardly traversed by her and Giulio. I ask her what she thinks was the reason that the leading did not work out properly. She doesn't know and assumes that Giulio simply did not react to her because he doesn´t take her seriously. She laughs, but is actually sad and disappointed. I give her the feedback that the actual problem is her lack of self-confidence. From her indicated movements, one can deduce that she knows when it would be right to give Giulio the signal to turn. But because she does not trust herself, because she does not take herself seriously, she indicates the signals only half-heartedly, instead of giving Giulio decisive, clear signals. In short: "Your problem is not a lack of skills, but a lack of self-confidence. Step forward confidently next time, trust yourself to carry out a movement, give clear signals!" Participant 2 starts the exercise again, and she manages to strive more clearly forward, not just to indicate movements, but to carry them out clearly to the end. Thereby she finally succeeds in leading Giulio confidently through the imagined triangle. ◀

Hence, the actual work with the dog build upon the initially failed exercises. The first correction of one's own mistakes, the first overcoming of insecurities usually give the participant a boost. The motivation to gradually approach more difficult exercises with the dog increases. We often observe a rapid increase in self-confidence and the feeling of self-efficacy.

▶ **Important!** More significant than the successes are the failed exercises with the dog.

5.2.2.5 Setbacks to Make Progress

The further sessions serve to expand self-confidence by gradually increasing the difficulty level of the exercises. It can also happen that participants have to face setbacks in the course of the exercises. This is part of the process.

Example: Taking Steps Back to Make Progress

Participant 2, after completing several leadership trainings with Giulio, has now developed her leadership skills to the point where she can confidently guide Giulio through a slalom course and even work with him partially off-leash. She arrives at the sessions excited. Her mood is good, she is relaxed and says of herself that she feels internally secure when she works with Giulio.

At the beginning of the session, she leads Giulio on a leash to the training area. She is in good spirits and talkative, and therefore distracted. She does not notice that she is not in touch with Giulio, that she and Giulio are not "in contact".[10] As a result, he turns to himself and sends signals to go in the other direction—probably following an interesting scent. For Participant 2, this happens completely unexpectedly, so she does not see his turn coming, and the leash suddenly tightens. She stops and doesn't know what to do. This has never happened to her before. Giulio always went straight to the training area. Due to the unexpected situation, Participant 2 falls back into her pattern of insecurity and not taking herself seriously. She says questioningly "Giulio come..", stands there uncertainly, laughs, looks questioningly to me. The friendly clarity with which she confidently guided Giulio through the slalom in the last session is blown away. Through my questions ("What do you want from Giulio at the moment? What signals does he need from you?") and assistance ("Stand up internally again. Forget that Giulio just surprised you with his behavior. Recall what you already know and can do to lead Giulio.") Participant 2 can finally address Giulio in

---

[10] I like to use the phrase "having the dog in contact". This means being attentive to the dog and perceiving that he is also attentive to me. This contact with the dog does not always have to be an active process externally (i.e., through direct eye contact or addressing the dog), it can also take place in silence. Every dog owner probably knows what this means. The mutual concentration on each other; the feeling that I have the dog with me, that we are doing something together.

a friendly and confident manner with a clear "Come" and at the same time go deter-
minedly in the direction she wants, so that Giulio follows her to the training area. We
use this situation to discuss the relevance of concentration and constructive handling
of "unplanned" events. After the conversation, Participant 2 finds her way back to her
learned self-confident behaviors and maintains a certain humility, which keeps her
attentive and focused before, during, and after the actual exercises with Giulio. ◄

The good thing about such setbacks is that we can use them in training to consolidate the
skills. The example of Participant 2 points out two general aspects that are relevant in the
course of dog leadership training and in the course of any developmental process:

- We always do well to maintain a certain humility (see Table 5.4) and to not take success (for example, of an exercise) for granted. This keeps us focused and concentrated, which in turn is the basic prerequisite for further success.
- We can only speak of having learned something when we can recall what we have
  learned in new, unforeseen situations.

Hence, as soon as we are at a point in training where the participants start to feel more
confident, it is advantageous if situations occur that challenge this still somewhat fragile
self-confidence. Only by facing challenges the self-confidence is stabilized.

▶   **Important!** By challenging what has been learned, self-confidence is stabi-
      lized in the long term.

5.2.2.6 Conclusion of the Self-Confidence Training

When the participant reaches the point where they can adequately handle the dog even
in difficult situations and thus react with self-confidence, we have reached our journey's
goal: In the dog's eyes, the participant is a "leadership personality", the participant is
self-confident towards the dog.

Example: Conclusion of the Self-Confidence Training

Participant 2 has arrived at the end of the leadership training, it is the tenth session.
Previously, we had practiced leading without a leash in increasingly difficult situations.
Today, the conclusion takes place with a course. The course consists of four closely
spaced pylons, a subsequent 50 cm high obstacle, and a mat. Participant 2 is supposed
to guide Giulio through the pylons in a slalom, have him jump over the obstacle, and
then have him lie down directly on the mat. The challenge for Participant 2 is the rapid
change of behavior she shows. In the slalom, she should guide Giulio calmly and con-
centratedly, indicate the necessary changes of direction with clear gestures, and walk
around the pylons at a slow pace with him. Coming out of the slalom, she should
immediately activate Giulio through a dynamic voice and body language, so that he

can jump high enough over the obstacle. Immediately afterwards, it is up to Participant 2 to take out the dynamics and regulate Giulio immediately into relaxation, so that he lies down relaxed on the mat. She must play with her external impact, switch from dynamics to calm and vice versa, thus have a fine sense for her effect and at the same time always have the situation under control. Participant 2 is highly motivated. We had practiced the individual components of the course in the previous session, she happily engages in the now assembled course. She is curious whether she will succeed and at the same time shows a relaxed serenity: "Hey, even if it doesn't work out perfectly, the most important thing is that Giulio and I are having fun!"

On the first run, Giulio skips a pylon because Participant 2 left too little space between herself and the pylon. After skipping the one pylon, she doesn't stop, but pulls through the course with Giulio as if nothing had happened—just as I had taught her in the previous sessions. If something doesn't work out, don't let it unsettle you, just keep going casually! Analysis is done after the exercise. She realizes herself that she needs to give Giulio more space in the slalom. After a petting break, she starts the course again with Giulio. She implements everything confidently, which keeps Giulio always motivated to follow her instructions. Participant 2 concludes her leadership training with a successfully mastered course, highly delighted. What pleased me most was her statement in the debriefing: "It was great that everything worked out so perfectly, but I am now confident enough that it probably wouldn't have bothered me if it had worked out less well." ◄

Once the self-confidence training is completed in terms of content, the final points are the closing discussion and the farewell. The closing discussion serves to summarize the training, to look back at the beginning and the hurdles taken in the course, and to appreciate the participant's development. I mentally go back with the participant to the first session and his initial behavior and contrast these with the development that has taken place and the now higher self-confidence. Some participants appreciate it if we write down the achieved changes together, and the participant can then take the written record with them. Others do not need or want this. I leave it up to the participant whether they want to take something written with them. Many participants want a souvenir photo of themselves with the dog at the end (or even during the self-confidence training), which I am of course happy to facilitate. Such a photo is more than a memory of a good time with the dog. It is used by many participants as a reminder of the contents of the self-confidence training. I know from some that they stamp this picture and hang it next to their PC or on refrigerator or even mirror to remind themselves daily of what they have accomplished and learned.

Moreover, a photo can make it easier for some participants to say goodbye to the dog at the end of the training. This farewell is not always easy and should not happen suddenly, but rather be prepared. Small rituals and gestures can make saying goodbye easier. For example, a small farewell gift for the dog can lead the participant to mentally prepare for the farewell from the dog in advance of the last session and make them better accept this step. Going into the forest and looking for a stick for the dog to chew or fetch is something I often recommend. The participant has to spend a little time and think about which stick is the right one for the dog. When he then gives the stick to the dog and the dog enthusiastically starts chewing on it, the session ends on a joyful note. The participant also leaves with the feeling of having left something of themselves to the dog.[11]

5.3   Potential Difficulties in Dog-Assisted Self-Confidence Training

The therapist has various aspects to consider and must respond to unforeseen events in a timely and constructive manner—always with the individual goal of the participant in mind. To work in the field of animal-assisted therapy is, hence, complex work. Even though we always have a similar goal in mind, namely the increase in self-confidence, each session with each participant is different, each session is a challenge for me as a therapist.

However, I can look back on work with participants who were particularly challenging for me, which means they made me face difficulties. I would like to introduce four categories of difficulties that I have encountered in the context of dog-assisted self-confidence training, and at the same time provide suggestions for dealing with these difficulties.

5.3.1   Participant Processes Feedback as Damaging to Self-Worth

A not infrequently occurring difficulty is the situation where a participant experiences the instructions and feedback from me as damaging to their self-worth. This is the case, in my experience, when the participant has low self-esteem and at the same time perceives their ability to establish good contact with dogs, or animals in general, as stabilizing factor of their self-worth. The background for this can be, for example, that the participant has repeatedly had very bad (or even traumatic) experiences with other people, or that they feel lonely in everyday life and reduce this feeling of loneliness having contact to animals (see Stanley et al., 2014). Since we work on the participant's relation-

---

[11] Sometimes you can't prevent participants from bringing a gift for the dog at the end. However, for professional ethical reasons, it is important that participants are not encouraged to bring a purchased toy or the like for the dog. For participants who would like to bring something for the dog, I recommend the above suggestion of bringing a stick or pine cone they have collected themselves. If their dog is not a "stick fan", they can also suggest bringing a piece of cheese or a carrot or another simple treat for the dog. Here too, it is important to ensure that the participant is not encouraged to go out and buy expensive treats.

ship building in the context of animal-assisted self-confidence training, participants with this initial situation often have difficulties dealing with feedback from the dog or me.

Example: Participant Processes Feedback as Damaging to Self-Worth

Participant 4 has experienced many disappointments and injuries from people in the past. He is initially mistrustful of people and avoids close contacts. However, he loves dogs very much. At the beginning of the training, he describes how quickly he is always able to bound with dogs, that every dog likes him, and that he is a "dog person". However, Participant 4 has never had a dog of his own, and in the first spontaneous leading, he is very insecure. He keeps on pulling the leash, does not signal to Giulio what he wants from him, and does not praise Giulio. Giulio reacts with distance, keeps as far away from Participant 4 as possible, avoids eye contact. Participant 4 does not respond to my first subtle feedback, but instead talks again about his good contact with dogs, repeatedly emphasizing how well he can assess dogs, how much dogs like him. ◄

There is a significant discrepancy between Participant 4's self-assessment and his actual relationship competence in dealing with the dog. Since his competencies in dealing with dogs are a major part of his self-image and are relevant to his self-esteem, he tries to block out critical feedback. As a therapist, I am now faced with two possible risks in such situations: I express the critical feedback so clearly that the participant can no longer ignore it. Then he is likely to react either with the sudden termination of therapy or with psychological decompensation. Or I hold back with my feedback to avoid hurting the participant, which in turn leads to him enjoying the training but not changing anything and not learning anything. So what to do instead? In such a case open, and sensitive communication is needed at an early point.

Example: Dealing with a participant who experiences feedback as damaging to self-esteem

I sit down with Participant 4 after the first training session and first ask him about his well-being during and after the training. After we have discussed this, I say (approximately) the following: "As you told me last time, I experienced today that contact with dogs is a very important resource for you. As a "dog person", I can fully understand this—it's no different for me. And now I just wondered during the training how you feel about receiving feedback about your interaction with Giulio. Feedback can sometimes be critical. How does it feel to you when I criticize something?" Participant 4 does not initially respond directly to my question, he evades. So I ask again very directly: "Does it hurt you when I evaluate something about your behavior towards Giulio and make suggestions for improvement?". Participant 4 answers shamefully "A little." With this honest answer, we have created the basis to openly discuss the topic. With Participant 4, it is discussed that it is better for him to stop the self-confidence training, as the critical examination of his own behavior towards the dog scratches too much at his self-esteem and thus destabilizes him. As an alternative, he continues regular psychotherapy and additionally just walks dogs from the animal shelter. ◄

By having an open conversation, we were able to find a suitable solution for Participant 4 early on. In other cases, where contact with dogs is also relevant to participants' self-esteem, it may well be that the participants can still engage in self-confidence training. This varies greatly from individual to individual. In any case, it is necessary to have an early clarifying conversation with these participants and to address one's own perception carefully but openly.

5.3.2   Participant Does Not Develop Awareness of their Impact on the Dog

Another difficulty I occasionally encounter during training is the situation where the participant does not develop a sense of their impact on the dog. In such cases, it can happen that the participant is unable to engage in the analysis of their own behavior and instead attributes the dog's behavior to other factors.

Example: Participant has little sense of her impact

Participant 5 is a young woman with severe social difficulties and pronounced self-doubt. She also struggles with the initial simple exercises to lead Cleo confidently. Participant 5 walks slowly and hesitantly next to Cleo, withdraws in body language and lets Cleo take the lead, instead of appearing determined and active. When Cleo is thus a step ahead, Participant 5 slows down even more, sighs exasperatedly, and pulls on the leash. Cleo reacts for a brief moment, but is confused by the unclear messages and overtakes Participant 5 again after a short time. Cleo does not understand what is expected of her: on the one hand, she gets leash pressure, on the other hand, Participant 5 does not take the lead, but passively lags behind and practically forces Cleo into the leadership position. I interrupt the session and have a conversation with Participant 5. She sees no responsibility on her part—Cleo is simply difficult today. She cannot make sense of my feedback that she is not sending clear signals to Cleo, establishing too little positive contact, and overall appearing too passive. If anything, she believes she is "too nice" to Cleo, and Cleo then takes advantage of this. ◄

Similar to this example, it often happens in practice that participants are not aware of their external impact and, hence, initially don´t understand the feedback. In such a case, I have found working with video recordings to be helpful. If the participant agrees, I film sequences from the training and we watch them together afterwards.[12] The great advantage is that the participant can observe themselves from the outside. They see, for example, that they are indeed walking very slowly or hunched over, that their voice indeed sounds exasperated, or their reaction to the dog's behavior is indeed too sluggish. The dog's reactions can also be examined in detail again. Participants with distorted self-perception or participants who are stressed by the training and therefore less reflective at the moment, usually benefit greatly from working with video analyses. Often, it is then sufficient to work with video analysis in one or two sessions. Afterwards, the willingness to accept feedback and implement changes increases significantly, and work can continue without recordings.

5.3.3   Participant Pursues a Different Goal

The following situation has particularly challenged me at the beginning of my work as an animal-assisted therapist: The participant pursues a different goal than I do. My goal is to increase the participant's self-confidence through training with the dog. Sometimes it can happen that the participant superficially agrees to this goal, but internally actually pursues a different goal or wants to use the sessions for something else.

In my experience, these other interests or needs are usually:

- The participant primarily wants to provide themselves with closeness by having contact with the dog
- The participant wants to use the sessions to talk about their problems and worries

---

Example: Participant Pursues a Different Goal

Participant 6 is undergoing treatment for various mental impairments and is very unstable and repeatedly stands out due to strong emotional reactions and behaviors. At the third session of the dog-assisted self-confidence training she arrives in tears. She simply can't go on, she feels very bad. She expresses the desire to just spend time with Giulio. I agree, she pets Giulio, talks to him, plays with him. The shared time with the dog leads to a short-term improvement in her condition. In the further course of the self-confidence training, such situations occur repeatedly. The actual goal, to increase her self-confidence, increasingly fades into the background. ◄

The problem with such situations is that the therapist and participant are pursuing different things. There is no real collaboration. If a participant, who is also in psychotherapy, for example, feels the need to "speak out" during the self-confidence training, this

---

[12] I would like to emphasize again at this point for data protection reasons the importance of a written consent to create these film recordings and the subsequent deletion of the recordings.

is detrimental to both therapies. On the one hand, this takes away time for working on self-confidence, on the other hand, the participant addresses important issues in a setting where they cannot be resolved for various reasons. So, through his behavior, he avoids two things that are relevant to him: on the one hand, the (exhausting) work on his self-confidence and on the other hand, the (exhausting) solution to his problems within the framework of psychotherapy. Therefore, repeatedly addressing worries and burdens during self-confidence training should be stopped early on. To clarify: Of course, it is important at the beginning of the session to know how the participant is doing and what is currently occupying him. I always ask this at the beginning of the session. However, the exchange about this should be limited and not turn into a long conversation about the participant's burdens.

Another difficulty that can arise is that the participant has a strong need to provide himself with closeness through the dog. This is problematic because this need cannot be finally satisfied within the framework of animal-assisted therapy. If an unstable participant primarily pursues this interest, he will not reach the point where his need is satisfied. There is no solution, no conclusion, no enough. One would have to continue the animal-assisted therapy indefinitely. And yet, the participant would not feel better in the long term. The feelings of emptiness and not-enough closeness, as well as the need for symbiosis with another person or creature, would remain. The often-quoted saying by Confucius seems very appropriate to me in this context:

> "Give a man a fish and you feed him for a day. Teach a man to fish and you feed him for his lifetime."

This is nothing more than a plea for the support of independence and thus a fitting symbol for my attitude in animal-assisted therapy. In my opinion, it is not productive to give the person a good feeling in dealing with the dog and then send him home happy or at least comforted for the moment, but unchanged. I am always concerned with promoting the personal development of the participant.

This of course does not mean that the participant is not allowed to pet the dog and enjoy dealing with him. It simply means: As a therapist, I have to make sure that the participant and I are working towards the same goal, namely to increase his self-confidence. If the participant also enjoys the closeness to the dog and feels good—all the better.

But how to deal with the situation when I notice during the course that the participant has no real interest in increasing his self-confidence, but comes to the sessions for other reasons? Here, openly addressing one's own perception, the continuous reminder of the jointly agreed goals and focuses, or in some cases also the correction of the goal and focus, can help. In such situations, it is always important to explain in detail to the participant why one does not simply grant his wish and instead wants to work with him on his self-confidence. It is important that the participant understands that it is not about not wanting to grant him something. Instead, he should feel that the therapist is concerned with more, namely the long-term well-being of the participant.

Not all difficult situations can always be satisfactorily resolved within the framework of self-confidence training. However, the aim should be to try and search for individual solutions and compromises. If these are not feasible, one should not shy away from prematurely ending the therapy in the last resort. This should then—if possible—happen by mutual agreement and within the framework of a constructive final discussion.

5.3.4 Therapist Does Not Sufficiently Consider the Underlying Needs of the Participant

This last category of the potential difficulties presented here is perhaps the most interesting, as it can underlie other difficulties. Specifically, it is about the consequences for the therapy that can result from a lack of consideration of the participant's basic needs. Every person has certain basic needs that drive and guide them.

Regarding human basic needs, there have always been various psychological theories. Without being able to delve deeper into this complex topic at this point, I would like to highlight a category of needs that can be activated by contact with the therapy dog and in the setting of animal-assisted therapy and—if not recognized by the therapist—can lead to difficulties or misunderstandings. Namely: the need for attachment and the need for autonomy.

If the need for attachment is strongly pronounced in a person, they strive for a sense of belonging and are willing to restrict their own independence and freedom for it. This can lead to a lack of self-reliance or difficulties in making independent decisions and taking responsibility. On the other hand, a person whose need for autonomy is very high strives for independence and self-realization. Here, risks such as reduced relationships, inhibitions about asking other people for help, or feelings of loneliness exist. And in connection with the different needs, there are also different fears. For example, someone who has a very high need for attachment may fear loneliness and rejection. Someone with a high need for autonomy, on the other hand, may fear the loss of their independence and freedom.

What does this mean for animal-assisted therapy? If a participant has a high need for attachment or autonomy, these needs are usually activated in their relationships. And since animal-assisted therapy is primarily relationship work, the relationship with the dog or the therapist may activate these needs or the fears associated with them in the participant. If the therapist is not adequately prepared for this, it can lead to misunderstandings and conflicts in the therapy.

> **Example: Possible Misunderstandings Due to Lack of Consideration for Basic Participant Needs**
>
> Participant 7 came into the animal-assisted therapy with skepticism at the beginning. It couldn't be that hard to lead a dog, besides, the dogs do this every day, it's all auto-

mated by now [first possible misunderstanding]. I expressed understanding for this view of the participant and suggested that we do the introduction and a trial session (with the option to end the session at any time on his part) and then he decides for himself whether he wants to continue the therapy or not. Participant 7 was comfortable with this option, slowly engaged with the content and topics, and then decided to carry out the animal-assisted therapy. In the first three sessions, Participant 7 was late each time [second possible misunderstanding]. I did not question this, but let him have his way. From the fourth session on, he was always on time. Towards the end of the therapy, Participant 7 repeatedly brought up the impending farewell from Toni [third possible misunderstanding] on the sidelines of the sessions. Participant 7 had by now built a good relationship with Toni and it was noticeable that the farewell made him sad. This phase of therapy offered the opportunity to speak generally and openly about his handling of farewells, relationship design, and related fears.

Analysis: Participant 7 showed a high need for autonomy from the beginning. If the therapist does not recognize this as such, it can lead to various misunderstandings between the participant and the therapist over time. The *first possible misunderstanding* in this case would have been to misinterpret the initial skepticism of the participant as disinterest or devaluation. Rather, the skepticism was a protective mechanism due to the fear of too intense bonding. Under no circumstances should a confrontational approach be taken here. Instead, the therapist should give the participant the feeling of having space and freedom of decision. The *second possible misunderstanding* was the lateness. Participant 7 was here (consciously or unconsciously) expressing his need for autonomy and at the same time testing the resilience of the therapeutic relationship. If the participant is otherwise reliable and the lateness remains within reasonable limits, it may be useful to initially allow this as a concession to the participant's need for autonomy and to observe it over time. The *third possible misunderstanding* lies in dealing with the participant's subtle opening at the end. By discussing the farewell from Toni, he indirectly addressed his fear of attachment. If the therapist confronts the tentative statements too confrontationally, the participant may recoil. If, on the other hand, the therapist overlooks the participant's remarks, he misses an important opportunity in therapy. As so often, it is the golden mean that leads further here: respond to the statements, but subtly and step by step. ◄

At this point, it becomes clear how important a solid education and therapeutic experience are in order to work effectively and appropriately within the field of animal-assisted therapy.

In addition, regarding the needs of the participants:

* The therapist should give the participant space and rather observe and understand their behavior for a longer period of time than react quickly and spontaneously.
* The participant should be accompanied *at their individual pace*.
* Under no circumstances should the participant be confronted analytically with their presumed needs and fears! Deeper conversations in this regard are only possible on

the basis of a *resilient therapeutic relationship* and require, as mentioned, a solid basic education and experience.

5.4 Summary of the Key Aspects of Dog-Assisted Self-Confidence Training

At this point, I would like to summarize the key maxims of my concept of dog-assisted self-confidence training or my general understanding of animal-assisted therapy:

Animal-assisted therapy should serve to enhance the well-being of humans and the well-being of the therapy companion animal. The animal must not be seen as a means to an end, but must be taken seriously in its own interests and needs (see Sect. 2.3). Adopting an animal from animal welfare is a good basis for this (see Sect. 3.2.2). Because the *decision to adopt a dog instead of buying one* means a second chance in life for the individual dog. And it is not to be underestimated what this decision means for the position of the whole species in human society. Dogs are not reduced to their pedigree or their possibly exclusive origin, but are seen as individuals. Every dog, regardless of its breed, deserves a good life. The more people take this into account and consistently adopt dogs from animal welfare instead of buying them, the better the general situation of the dogs in our society will be.

Following the adoption of the dog, a *slow and positive training*, which recognizes and promotes the individuality and authenticity of the animal, as well as an *animal-friendly planning and implementation of the animal-assisted therapy* should naturally follow (see Chap. 3).

For the therapy, the main rule is: The well-being of the therapy companion animal takes precedence over all other goals and needs—be they one's own, those of the participant or those of the institution in which one works (see Sect. 6.1). This may lead to the need to make *unpopular decisions in favor of the animal* (see Sect. 3.5). And it applies: The *relationship* between the participant and the therapy companion animal is always more important than the performance, success or completion of an exercise or task (see Sect. 5.2.2).

In addition to the *necessity of broad dog and animal experience*, the basic prerequisite for animal-assisted therapy must be a *solid education* as well as sufficient experience in the therapeutic field.

Furthermore, for the effectiveness of animal-assisted therapy, it is important to recognize the *needs of the participant that stand behind the wishes and expectations* towards the animal and the animal-assisted therapy (see Sect. 5.3.4). Thus, the participant may primarily express a wish or have certain expectations. If these are simply fulfilled, one may satisfy the participant for the moment, but not achieve sustainable therapy success. Instead, it is central to the success of therapy to recognize what stands behind a statement, a wish or a behavior and to pick this up therapeutically, to make it understandable for the participant and possibly to work on it. In good animal-assisted therapy, the therapist and participant always work towards *the same goal* (see Sect. 5.3.3).

References

Albuquerque, N., Guo, K., Wilkinson, A., & Savalli, C. (2016). Dogs recognize dog and human emotions. *Biology Letters, 12*(1), 20150883. https://doi.org/10.1098/rsbl..2015.0883.

Buttner, A., Thompson, B., Strasser, R., & Santo, J. (2015). Evidence for a synchronization of hormonal states between humans and dogs during competition. *Physiology & Behavior, 147*, 54–62.

Campbell-Meiklejohn, D., Simonsen, A., Frith, C. D., & Daw, N. D. (2017). Independent neural computation of value from other people's confidence. *The Journal of Neuroscience, 37*(3), 673–684.

Collins, J. (2001). *Good to great. Why some companies make the leap... and others don't*. Random House Business Books.

D'Aniello, B., Semin, G. R., Alterisio, A., Aria, M., & Scandurra, A. (2018). Interspecies transmission of emotional information via chemosignals: From humans to dogs (canis lupus familiaris). *Animal Cognition, 21*(1), 67–78.

Fiedler, P., & Marwitz, M. (2016). Selbstunsichere und ängstlich-vermeidende Persönlichkeitsstörungen. *PSYCH up2date, 10*. https://doi.org/10.1055/s-0042-103824. Accessed: 9. July 2019.

Güroff, E. (2018). *Das Training sozialer Kompetenzen (TSK) in der stationären Praxis*. Klett-Cotta.

Lehenbauer, M. (2012). Primäre Prävention sozialer Ängste. Abgerufen am 09.07.2019 von urn:nbn:at:at-ubw:1-29172.62121.741560-8.

Mörtl, K., Epple, N., Rothermund, E., & Wietersheim, J. (2008). Gruppen—zwischen—Räume(n)—Eine qualitative Studie zum therapeutischen Transfer zwischen Tagesklinik und Zuhause. *Gruppenpsychotherapie und Gruppendynamik, 44*, 110–134.

Müller, C. A., Schmitt, K., Barber, A. L., & Huber, L. (2015). Dogs can discriminate emotional expressions of human faces. *Current Biology, 25*, 601–605.

O'Farrell, V. (1997). Owners attitudes and dog behavoir problems. *Applied Animal Behavior Science, 52*(3–4), 205–213.

Schöberl, I., Wedl, M., Beetz, A., & Kortschal, K. (2017). Psychobiological factors affecting cortisol variability in human-dogs dyads. *Plos One*. https://doi.org/10.1371/journal.pone.0170707.

Stanley, I. H., Conwell, Y., Bowen, C., & Van Orden, K. A. (2014). Pet ownership may attenuate loneliness among adult primary care patients who live alone. *Aging & Mental Health, 18*(3), 394–399.

Sundman, A. S., Van Poucke, E., Svensson Holm, A. C., Faresjö, A., Theodorsson, E., & Roth, L. S. (2019). Long-term stress levels are synchronized in dogs and their owners. *Scientific Reports, 9*(7391), 1–7.

Wischall-Wagner, A. (2019). *Entspannter Mensch—entspannter Hund ... so glückt das Zusammenleben wie von selbst*. Gräfe & Unzer.

Preparing the Dogs for their Deployment

Contents

Abstract

An entire book would be necessary to fully depict the training of dogs from animal welfare in preparation for their later use as therapy companion dogs. Therefore, this chapter can only provide a very general overview of some important aspects of training and preparing therapy companion dogs from animal welfare. Initially, this chapter is about the basic attitude in training, with which one should approach their dog and the training. Subsequently, it deals with the handling and unlearning of unwanted behaviors that dogs from animal welfare can bring along. I illustrate this using the specific example of my own dogs. Finally, some aspects of training in preparation for the use of dogs in therapy are described.

Supplementary Information The online version contains supplementary material available at https://doi.org/10.1007/978-3-662-67965-4_6. The videos can be accessed individually by clicking the DOI link in the accompanying figure caption or by scanning this link with the SN More Media App.

6.1   Basic Attitude

No other aspect determines the course, the feelings of human and dog during training, and the success of the training as much as the basic attitude that the human has towards themselves and the dog, and thus towards the training.

The best basis for sustainable and positive training is the following ultimate goal: *Human and dog should enjoy the training and become happier in the long term through the training.*

If this attitude is firmly anchored internally, then it leads to:

- gentle and positive training methods being used,
- understanding that a good relationship with the dog is more important than quick success
- a treatment of the dog as an individual and partner

It also includes a relaxed approach to one's own mistakes and the dog's mistakes. In this context, I advocate for serenity and humor in dealing with failure and mistakes (see Fig. 6.1). Humor carries you through difficult situations, connects human and dog, broadens the view, and makes us look for constructive ways instead of striving for success.

Fig. 6.1 Not everything works out right away in training—like here with leash guidance. Humor carries through these situations and maintains motivation

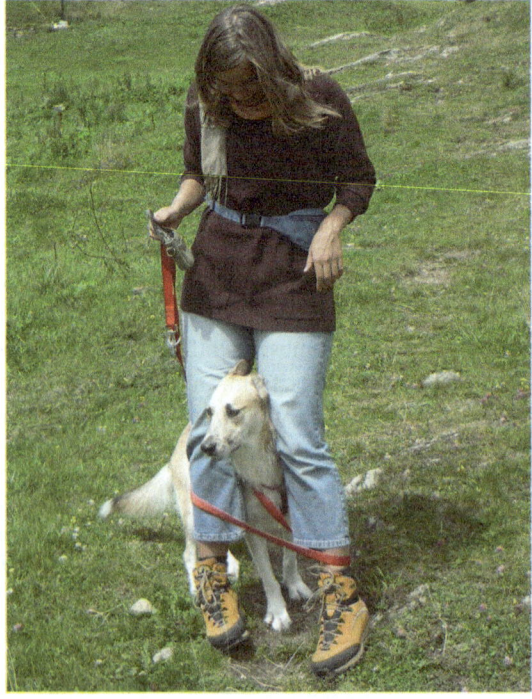

A benevolent and humorous attitude, where the joy of training and the long-term increase in the well-being of the human-dog team are in the foreground, should be the basis of the training.

Sometimes it is necessary for the development of this attitude to free oneself from one's own expectations regarding perfection and comparison with others. Because one thing should be clear: Every dog and every human and thus every human-dog team is unique. Every dog owner faces different challenges with their dog, lives in different life circumstances, brings different life experiences, and has different life goals. So comparing or even measuring oneself with other human-dog teams is nonsensical. Instead of striving for what others succeed in, the focus should always be on creating and maintaining a thoroughly positive relationship with one's own dog. The positive relationship with one's own dog and the increase in mutual well-being through training are fundamental for everything else and should always be in the foreground even in advanced training.

▶ **Important!** Every dog and every human and thus every human-dog team is unique. Every dog owner faces different challenges with their dog, lives in different life circumstances, brings different life experiences, and has different life goals. Therefore, the focus in training should never be on comparing with other dogs or other human-dog teams, but should always be directed at oneself and one's own dog. The ultimate goals of the training are the development and maintenance of a thoroughly positive relationship with the dog and the increase in mutual well-being.

This attitude is particularly central for later therapeutic work. Animal-assisted therapy, as outlined in the previous chapters, is primarily relationship work. The participant reflects and changes in the relationship with the dog. The therapeutic work is based on the relationship between the therapist and the therapy dog. The relationship is the basis of this therapy and is always at the center. Thus, the attitude of putting the relationship with the dog above success, performance, and other technical factors is an essential basis of animal-assisted therapy.

6.2   Specifics of Training Dogs from Animal Welfare

If we compare the training of rescued dogs with the training of dogs with unburdened origin and socialization, there are two possible differences. These concern the *duration of training* and the *difficulty level of training*. Thus, the training of a dog from a rescue can take longer and can be more difficult. Here, the term "can" is explicitly used. Just because a dog comes from a breeder and comes to its new people as a puppy, does not mean that its training is easy and quick. Because:

"There is no such thing as puppy training that educates your dog from the beginning in such a way that nothing needs to be practiced or explained anew for the next 15 years. Or do you know of such a kindergarten?" (Wischall-Wagner, p. 48)

And at the same time, it also applies: Just because a dog has lived in an animal shelter for a while or was born on the street, does not mean that its training is automatically lengthy and difficult. However, I do say that the training of rescued dogs can take longer and can be more complex because the dog's prior experiences may have shaped him in such a way that, for example, additional work on already learned behaviors is necessary.

6.2.1 Longer Duration and Higher Difficulty Level of Training

The training of a dog from a rescue can therefore take longer or be more complex due to several factors. First, there is the dog's acclimatization phase, which can take longer and pose challenges to people due to the dog's respective prior experiences. In addition, the dog must not only be taught new behaviors necessary for its later use, but often unwanted behaviors must also be unlearned.

6.2.1.1 Adjustment Phase

When a dog is adopted from an animal shelter, it must first settle into its new family and their lifestyle. This means that the dog has to adapt to new routines, new environments, new people, and new rules. This process sometimes runs more quickly and smoothly, sometimes more slowly and more difficult, as it depends on various factors—such as the individual character of the dog, its past history, the specific everyday conditions, and the experience, time, and patience of the human, as well as the specific everyday conditions. In any case, it takes time for the dog to settle into its new home, getting used to the new routines and the new people around it, and feeling safe and comfortable. At this point, it is not yet possible to think about real training or even preparation for work as a therapy companion dog.

"[The dog] moves into a completely new living space. How would you feel if you were suddenly dropped off on Mars with a UFO from one day to the next? [...] The solution here, as with many physical laws, lies in space and time" (Wischall-Wagner, 2019, p. 46).

So, patience must be shown towards the dog. Therefore, time and space are the most important keywords in the dog's adjustment phase.

In addition, this first phase of living together is about jointly managing mundane everyday situations. Perhaps the dog also needs to be made "suitable for everyday life"—not a few dogs with somewhat longer fur need a visit to the dog groomer or at least a thorough bath after their time in the animal shelter (see Fig. 6.2). The dog also needs to get used to new food and new feeding times. Likewise, its digestion must adjust to this new diet.

Fig. 6.2 Cleo needs a thorough wash after her adoption from the animal shelter

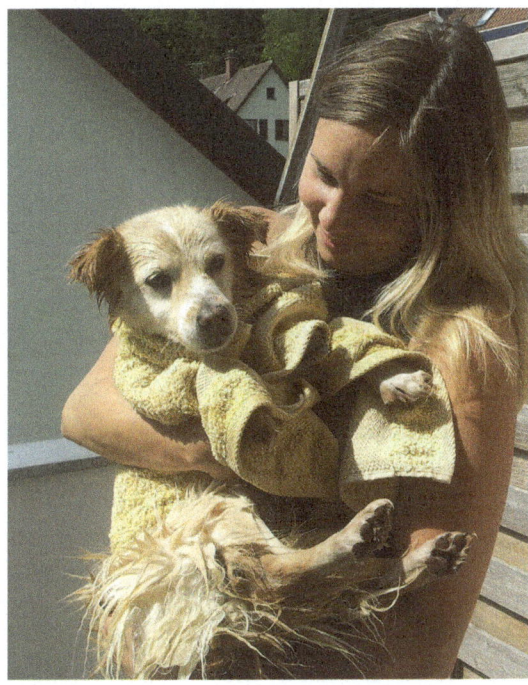

In short: These are very basic things that are initially important, and it may be that this adjustment phase takes a longer period of time. In addition to *giving time and space, optimism* is also a helpful inner attitude. Because anyone who lets themselves be discouraged by possible difficulties during this time or even starts to build pressure slows down the process.

Example: The adjustment period is not always easy

When Giulio joined the family, he was—as already mentioned elsewhere—far from being a pleasant family dog. He was kind and approachable, but showed some unpleasant behaviors. On his first day, for example, he had a hard time climbing the stairs in the house. Not because he had physical problems, but because he had never seen a staircase in his entire life, let alone walked up or down one. When he finally arrived upstairs with difficulty, Giulio suddenly stood in the middle of the dining table a few minutes later. He had jumped onto the dining table from a standing position and stood—proud and upright—in the middle of the table. He had only lived in his monotonous box so far, and a house with stairs, tables, and all the other new things were completely new territory for Giulio. Accordingly, in the first few weeks, all the rules that seem normal to us in dealing with these things had to be learned by him. The adjustment period can be a challenge for both dog and human and take time. ◄

6.2.1.2 Untraining Undesirable Behavior

The next reason why training with a dog from an animal shelter can take longer and be more challenging is that the dogs—due to their previous experiences—can bring certain unwanted behaviors. For example, they may have learned to be responsible for their own safety and food through living on the streets. Accordingly, such dogs may continue to independently search for food and eat things they find along the way after their adoption. Or the dog may have had bad experiences with other dogs in the shelter and therefore react fearfully or aggressively to other dogs. Such or other unwanted behaviors then need to be untrained, which can take a while.

Due to their individual history, each of my dogs also brought certain unwanted behaviors at the beginning.

6.2.1.2.1 Giulio: Untraining a Variety of Different Unwanted Behaviors

As described elsewhere (see Sect. 1.3.2), Giulio had by far the most difficult start in life of my three current dogs. Accordingly, the unwanted behaviors he initially exhibited were quite diverse (see Table 6.1). Of these behaviors, pulling on the leash and stereotypical licking behavior were relatively quickly trained out. Thus, everything in his life changed through adoption. Instead of sitting alone in the barren box, he now went for long, intensive walks several times a day and was mentally challenged for the first time in his life through family life and daily training sessions. This physical and mental exertion lowered his overall energy level and increasingly allowed him to relax, which automatically reduced the behaviors that were due to a high basic tension.

Table 6.1 Unwanted behaviors of the dogs at the beginning of their training

Dog	Unwanted Behavior	Training
Giulio	Hunting Behavior	• Recall training (outdoors) • Acclimatization to small animals (indoors)
	Stereotypical Licking	• Increase general ability to relax • Exertion through physical activity and mental stimulation
	Fear-induced aggressive behavior towards other dogs	• Desensitization and counterconditioning
	Strong Pulling on the Leash	• Leash training
Cleo	Eating from the Street	• Introduce "Stop" and "Take" commands
Toni	Strong Pulling on the Leash	• Leash training
	Hunting Behavior	• Recall training (outdoors) • Acclimatization to small animals (indoors)
	Excessive Greeting and Jumping Up	• Behavior extinction through ignoring

In addition to this, I conducted leash training with him to counteract pulling on the leash: As soon as Giulio pulled, I would stop. When he came back, the leash would loosen and the reward was to continue walking. This is quite a tedious undertaking at the beginning, as it feels like you are standing more than walking. But once the dog understands that he gets two pleasant things (namely a loose leash and forward movement) when he walks considerately and relaxed on the leash, this, in my experience, becomes particularly ingrained in the dog.

The hunting behavior was reduced in the house through successive acclimatization to the small animals (see Fig. 6.3) and during walks through recall training and work with the trailing leash. In the house, Giulio quickly established the so-called *castle peace*—that is, peaceful interaction with everyone who is considered part of the family.

After a short time, the small animals thus became part of the pack. As soon as Giulio comes home, his first stop is by the rabbits and guinea pigs. He greets them by bringing his snout close to their faces. Most of the time, the rabbits respond by standing on their hind legs and also touching him with their snouts. Thus, my dogs, rabbits, and guinea pigs not only live in the same household, but they live together and enjoy each other's company. Cleo even sleeps and rests with the rabbits (see Fig. 6.4).

If the dog's hunting behavior is very pronounced at the beginning, a water pistol can be used for help. Although I am reluctant to work with punishment or unpleasant meth-

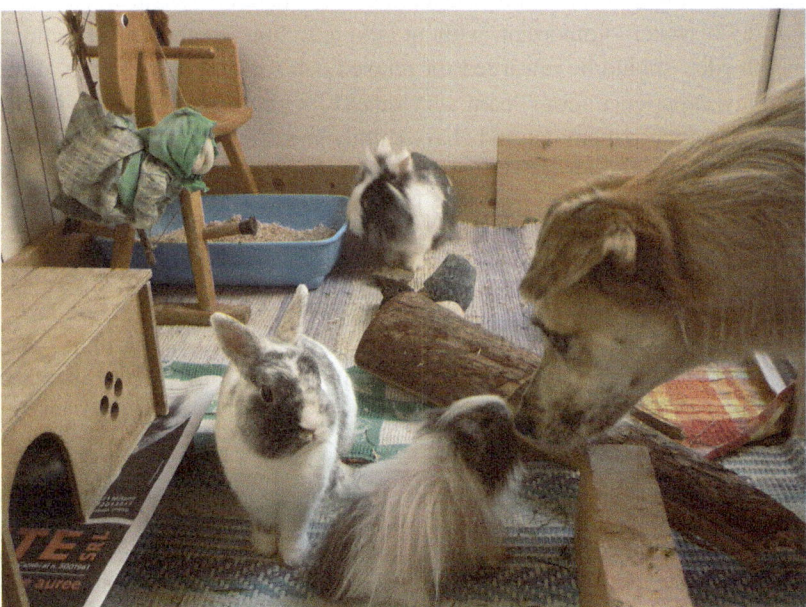

Fig. 6.3 Hunting behavior eliminated through training: Giulio lives peacefully with the rabbits and guinea pigs

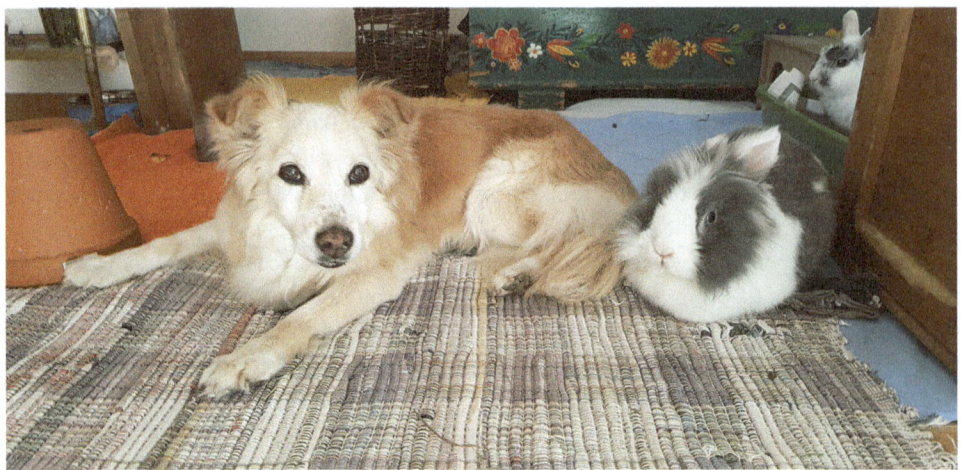

Fig. 6.4 Living together—Cleo and Alice enjoy resting together

ods, this is an exception as it is about enabling safe and stress-free coexistence. Often it is not necessary, but there are cases where the hunting behavior is very pronounced, and then the use of a water pistol is an effective and quick-acting method (if used correctly, which applies to all methods). It works in a few words as follows: If the dog fixates the small animal with his gaze (this is the beginning of the behavior chain when hunting), he gets a short jet of water—important: without talking to him or otherwise reacting. At the same time, the dog should be rewarded for relaxed behavior in the presence of the small animals. In my experience, dogs learn very quickly with this not to fixate on the small animals and not to harm them, but to behave calmly and relaxed in their presence.

Excursion: Some Important Terms from Dog Training
Impulse Control
= "the restraint (inhibition), the attenuated response to a suddenly occurring stimulus in connection with the ability to endure frustration" (Ullrich, 2016, p. 18)
  Classical Conditioning
= a stimulus (example: presence of another dog), which is associated with a certain event (example: being threatened, being bitten). The originally neutral stimulus thereby triggers a certain expectation or emotion (example: fear) and thus a certain behavior (example: defense through aggressive behavior) in the future.
  Counterconditioning
= a stimulus (example: presence of another dog), which previously triggered a certain behavior (example: defense through aggressive behavior), is linked through classical conditioning to a new expectation and thus a new behavior (example: waiting for treats), which is incompatible with the previous behavior. As a result, the newly learned behavior (example: waiting for treats) is used to respond to the stimulus (example: presence of another dog), leading to an inhibition or extinction of the previous behavior (example: defense through aggressive behavior).
  Desensitization

= Gradual confrontation or approach to a fear-inducing stimulus (example: presence of another dog), so that the fear diminishes over time

Training Giulio to stop hunting behavior during walks took significantly longer than getting him used to small animals in the home environment. Reducing hunting behavior in the open field is often challenging because chasing has a high self-rewarding character. This is especially true if the dog has ever had "success", i.e., caught or even killed an animal. Fortunately, this was not the case with Giulio. However, the training was not easy due to his initially generally low *impulse control*. It took many months before I could let Giulio roam freely without worries.

The necessary recall training with him was designed in such a way that Giulio learned to associate a certain whistle with the gift of a treat that is attractive to him (the attractiveness of a treat varies for many dogs over time, for Giulio at that time it was cooked beef, currently it is, for example, dried chicken). The association *whistle—super treat* is solidified in the course of a conditioning process through repetition—initially with the dog on a long leash, then gradually without a long leash and at increasing distances and increasingly under distraction—until it leads to a reliable recall signal. This takes longer

Fig. 6.5 Recall training Toni
with the help of Giulio
(▶ https://doi.org/10.1007/000-axj)

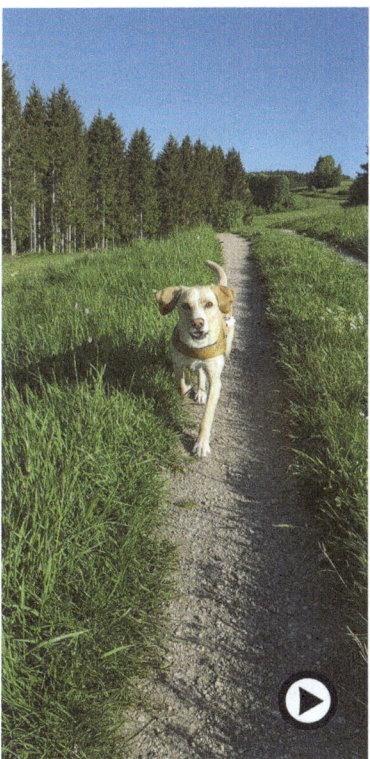

„Giulio, Toni!" and than a whistle

or shorter depending on the intensity of practice, depending on the dog and depending on the training environment. For example, it is easier to reliably recall the dog in a city park than in a forest area with a high presence of wildlife.

Training becomes easier if you can train the learning dog with the support of a dog that already reliably comes back. Thus, recall training with Toni became significantly easier for me, as Giulio is now a great support: I call the two of them, Giulio runs off to come back, and Toni follows Giulio. As a result, Toni learns to come back faster than if I were to train him alone (see Fig. 6.5).

Before I could, however, carry out the recall training with Giulio, we first had to overcome the biggest challenge, namely reducing Giulio's fear-induced aggressive behavior towards other dogs. At the beginning, Giulio could not tolerate any strange dog in his vicinity—and vicinity here means even seeing the dog from a distance. As soon as he spotted a point several hundred meters away that he recognized as a dog, he threw himself into the leash, barked and growled. The closer the dog, the more intense Giulio's reaction. Since I had always had very sociable dogs, i.e., dogs that got along wonderfully with every other dog, Giulio's behavior was very unusual for me. It therefore took some time until I found the right training method to reduce this behavior, namely *counterconditioning* and *desensitization*.

Specifically, the counterconditioning looked like this: As soon as Giulio and I spotted a dog in the distance, he received a treat. Always. Regardless of whether the dog was in the garden behind a fence, whether it was a puppy, whether it was a barking dog on television. Whenever a dog was somehow present, Giulio received a reward. And now comes the perhaps absurd sounding, but crucial point: he received the reward regardless of how he behaved! Many are initially surprised by this, because it seems to them that the dog will then rage even more in the future, as he was supposedly rewarded for it. But this is a misconception. We have to imagine that Giulio (due to the bite he suffered as a puppy—see Sect. 1.3.2) was afraid of other dogs and wanted to keep them at a distance through his fear-induced aggressive behavior. The treat creates a counterconditioning— so instead of the presence of another dog causing fear, Giulio associates the presence of another dog with the pleasant receipt of a treat. Instead of "Dog = Fear", Giulio is taught the connection "Dog = Joy (about the treat)".

The development of the new feeling towards the presence of another dog happens in steps. And this is where we come to desensitization. Giulio quickly learned to tolerate the distant dog well and to react to its presence with joyful anticipation of a treat. Now it was about gradually accepting more and more proximity to the other dog. The distance to the other dogs was gradually reduced, with Giulio's fear of the other dogs slowly becoming weaker and weaker.

It was a long journey, as Giulio's fear was pronounced and had solidified over the years. Moreover, not every dog encounter can be controlled—one turns a corner and unexpectedly runs into another dog, or a loose dog may suddenly approach. If this results in a threatening experience for the dog in training, it is a setback. But this is part of every training: there are advances, there are setbacks, it stagnates, one has doubts and yet continues, and one day persistence pays off, and the problems dissolve. Sometimes it's like a knot bursting.

And so it happened that Giulio was able to shed his unwanted behaviors so well that he has now been living with changing other dogs for many years without any problems (see Fig. 6.6). Giulio is the point of orientation for the other dogs. He gives them security, he is patient and friendly.

6.2.1.2.2 Cleo: Unlearning Eating from the Street

Cleo's only unwanted behavior was eating from the street. Otherwise, despite the fact that she had lived on the street for several years, she was completely easy to handle from the start and one of the fastest and easiest dogs to train that I have ever had. Her street eating was not only with earthworms (see Sect. 3.2), but with anything that seemed edible to her in the broadest sense. It was touching that she always wanted to share. For example, she once found a meatball and instead of eating it alone, she brought the meatball to me to share. The fact that I took it away from her was then a bitter disappointment for her. To reduce this behavior—which is potentially very dangerous, considering poison baits or dropped medications—I introduced the commands *Take* and *Stop*.

Take can be practiced well with feeding or in between with treats. The dog is made to wait with hand signals and command (*Wait*), so it should learn not to pounce on the food immediately. The waiting is resolved with the word *Take*. The command *Stop* is then associated with taking something out of the mouth. Once these signals are firmly established, they are used on walks when the dog is about to pick something up with its mouth to eat it. Ideally before picking it up, a clear *Stop* signals that the dog should not take it. Then, in exchange for the uneaten "treat" on the street, it gets a treat. This

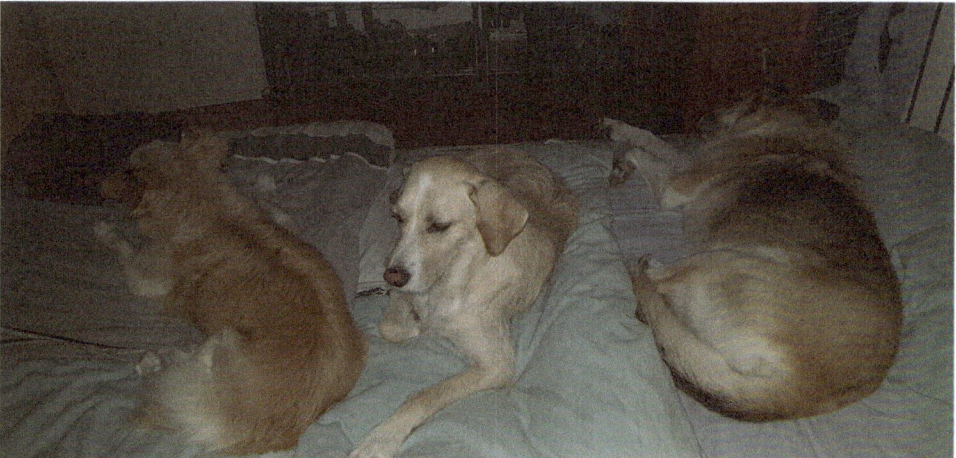

Fig. 6.6 Giulio (right) in relaxed proximity with other dogs—who would have ever dared to hope for this at the beginning!

should—accompanied by the command *Take*—be given. This way, the dog gets used to "reaching" only on command. Cleo was able to stop eating on the street on her own very quickly with this method.

6.2.1.2.3 Toni: Training to Reduce Excessive Greeting and Jumping Up

Toni brought along the unwanted behaviors of hunting behavior, strong pulling on the leash, and excessive greeting with jumping up. I will not go into more detail about training out the hunting behavior and the strong pulling on the leash, as the corresponding training has already been demonstrated using Giulio as an example. However, it should be noted again at this point that Toni's training is facilitated by the presence of Giulio (see Fig. 6.7). Giulio walks on a loose leash, comes when called, treats the rabbits and guinea pigs lovingly—all of this positively influences Toni and significantly shortens certain training processes.

Toni is a very intelligent and sociable dog. When I met him at the animal shelter, he was literally "hanging" on the kennel door—this was, as I recall, also the reason why he immediately stood out from the crowd of other dogs and drew my attention. With

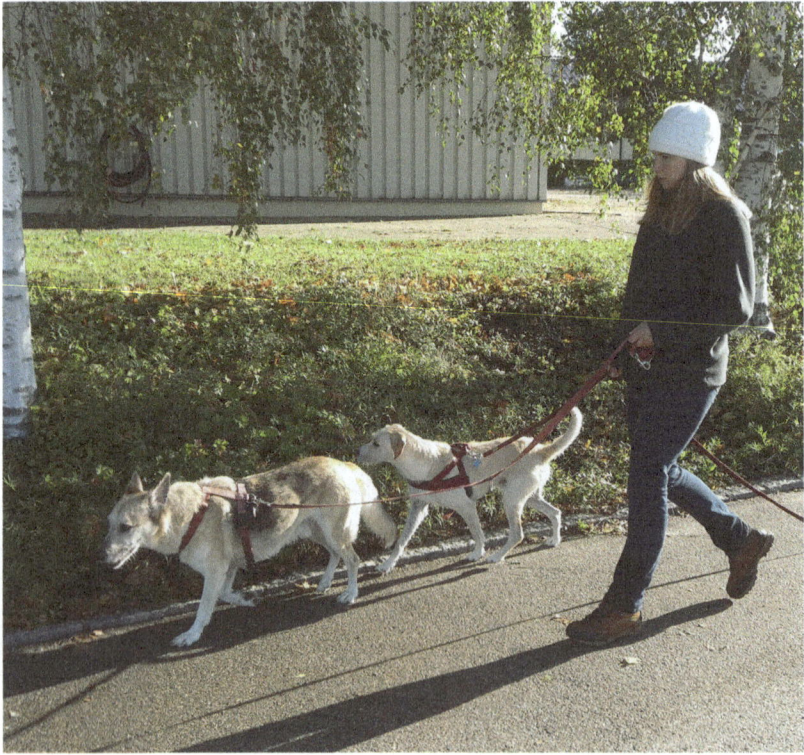

Fig. 6.7 Giulio as my co-trainer: When walking, Toni lines up behind Giulio, as Giulio walks on a loose leash, Toni becomes leash-trained almost by himself

plate-sized, kind eyes, he stood on his hind legs and paddled with his front legs up the wire door. He did not bark, as many dogs in the shelter do when visitors walk through the corridors, but fought for the attention of passers-by by jumping up and standing on his hind legs. He kept this strategy of making contact and gaining attention even after his adoption from the shelter. When someone he liked came to visit, he was over the moon and jumped up at them with all his might. This is actually a behavior that can usually be trained out of dogs quite easily. However, the behavior of some visitors presented me with not insignificant additional difficulties. Toni is not very big, so most people don't mind when he jumps up at them. And since many are touched by his openness and sociability, initially some acquaintances and strangers unintentionally encouraged the jumping up. "I don't mind!" was a common statement. Unfortunately, it is often forgotten that the dog therefore continues to "try his luck" with others, as he has success with jumping up with some people and does not consistently fail with this behavior. Implementing the concept of consistent ignoring and turning away when jumping up was therefore difficult. The dog should always be ignored by every person he jumps up at for this behavior. This means specifically that the jumping up is not responded to and physically turned away or turned away from. If the dog then approaches appropriately, he is greeted friendly. This eliminates jumping up as a behavior during greeting, as the dog learns that it does not lead him to his goal—namely, establishing positive contact with people.

This example of jumping up shows how important it often is to also involve the wider environment in the training. This is especially true when it comes to extinguishing an unwanted behavior. Because if the dog continues to be reinforced in his unwanted behavior, it is difficult to achieve a complete extinction of behavior. Instead, the dog will always "try his luck" again if he can hope to sometimes receive positive feedback for his behavior.

6.2.2 Personal Attitude

Adopting, acclimating, and later training and educating dogs from animal shelters may seem more demanding than getting a puppy from a breeder. However, it should not be forgotten that a puppy from a breeder also needs to be acclimated, educated, trained, and educated at home. And this can also bring challenges, depending on the character of the dog and especially the experience of the person.

The specific hurdles one will encounter in the further course when deciding on a dog are always uncertain. Therefore, personal attitude is all the more important.

If I assume that every hurdle and every difficulty is an opportunity for personal growth and development—both for me as a dog handler and for me as a person—then I can deal with them benevolently. Because not only in life, but also in dog training, it applies: "You can make lemonade out of every sour lemon. Sometimes you only recognize the opportunity or the lemonade in retrospect, you only realize in retrospect what something was ultimately good for" (Fiss-Quelle, 2016, p. 74).

If I also assume that I am primarily adopting a new family member and only second-arily wish to make a therapy companion dog out of him, then I can approach the training calmly. I have no internal pressure that the dog "must function". Because—and I cannot emphasize this enough—even if I choose the dog according to the previously described criteria (see Sect. 4.2), I have *no guarantee* that he will actually become a good therapy companion dog! And it should be clear: Whoever has brought a dog into his home is responsible for his life and well-being. And this regardless of whether he—as perhaps hoped and planned—can become a therapy companion dog or whether it turns out that he does not enjoy the work or is not suitable for other reasons. The dog is and remains a family member.

Understanding the dog as a family member and friend; approaching the training of the dog calmly, in a good mood and without pressure to succeed, and seeing emerging difficulties in training or everyday life as an opportunity for personal development—this is the advice I can give to anyone who wants to work with dogs (whether from animal shelters or not).

▶   **Important!** Those who want to live and perhaps also work with dogs should:

- Understand the dog as a family member and friend
- Approach the training of the dog calmly, in a good mood and without pressure to succeed
- Understand emerging difficulties in training or everyday life as an oppor-tunity for personal development

6.3   Training as a Therapy Companion Dog

Once the dog's unwanted behaviors have been eliminated, the dog can be prepared for its work as a therapy companion dog. Often, one (future) animal-assisted therapist is con-nected to a training institute for this, which means that their training and examination statutes are the guideline for the dog's training.

I instead train my dogs myself and describe here in broad terms what I personally pay attention to when training my dogs. However, it should be clear that the content of the training must be based on what you want to do with the dog later on, and what specific rules the respective examination or training institute or the institution with which you are working or want to work with in the future has.

In Sects. 1.3.3 and Chap. 3 I have outlined my fundamental attitudes and focuses in dealing with my animals and dogs both in training and during and after therapeutic work. Here, based on this, I describe the most important behaviors that my dogs learn for their use in therapy and self-confidence training.

6.3.1 Basics: Dog Reliably Responds to Basic Signals

As the basis of any further training, the dogs should know basic rules and signals that are relevant for living together with humans and for safety in everyday life. Some people refer to this as *basic obedience*, I call it the *basic rules of the game* in cohabitation between humans and dogs. This includes the following basics (listed with the respective signal word and hand sign):

It is important to mention that the unlearning of unwanted behaviors (see Sect. 6.2.1.2) and the learning of basic signals usually run parallel and merge into each other. For example, hunting behavior can only be stopped by training the recall signal, and some of the other signals must be learned in order to be able to unlearn certain unwanted behaviors. At the same time, the dog sometimes already has to have discarded certain behaviors in order to be able to learn certain signals (see Table 6.2). The unlearning of unwanted behaviors and the establishment of a reliable execution of signals merge into each other, mutually influence each other and are thus to be understood as a continuum.

Table 6.2 Basics

Signal word	Hand sign	Dog performs the following behavior
"Come"	Tap on leg with hand	Dog comes
Whistle (recall signal)	–	Dog comes (even from large distance and when distracted)
"Sit"	Raised index finger	Dog sits down
"Place"	Hand points to the lying place	Dog goes to his lying place
"Down"	Open hand with palm facing down goes towards the ground	Dog lies down
"Wait"	If dog should stop while running: - If visual contact exists: Open hand with palm facing the dog	Dog remains in his position
"Slow"	–	Dog slows his pace
"Go"	Sweeping arm movement	Dog is released from a previous signal (can continue walking, start running, and so on)
"Stop"	–	Dog interrupts an unwanted behavior
"Take"	Hand points to food/toy	Dog is allowed to take food or toy
"Search"	–	Dog uses eyes and nose to search for something
"It's okay"	Visible relaxation of body posture for the dog (conscious lowering of the shoulders, exhaling)	Dog relaxes

6.3.2   Training Necessary Behaviors for Therapy

What specific behaviors do I teach my dogs so that they can be used in my form of animal-assisted therapy? There are not many behaviors, because, as I said, my dog-assisted self-confidence training is about the participant receiving *honest and authentic feedback from the dog* and being able to reflect on their own behavior. So what do I train—beyond the basic and the elaborate reduction of unwanted behavior—with my dogs so that they can act as mirrors for the participants in therapy?

In preparing my future therapy companion dog, I focus on the following aspects:

- **Focus on Participant**: I teach the dog to have little or no contact with me during a therapy session and instead to focus on the participant
- **Authenticity:** I encourage the dog's authentic and individual reactions to human behaviors
- **Experience**: I accustom the dog to contact and cooperation with a wide variety of people in a wide variety of settings

In the nd these are only very few points, but building these comprehensively and appropriately for each dog is anything but trivial. It requires a good eye for the respective dog, continuous and tailored training, as well as high attention and presence in all shared everyday situations.

It should also be mentioned at this point that the training of a therapy companion dog is never really completed. Every contact with a participant affects the dog—hence, as explained in Sects. 3.6 and 3.7, the creation of balance and good design of breaks are so important for maintaining the mental health of the therapy companion dog. But even when observing breaks and creating a healthy balance, the dog's behavior is influenced by long-term patient or participant contact. I like to compare this influence of the participants on the dog to the steady, soft water drop that, over a long period of time, is still able to hollow out a hard stone. Therefore, it is also and especially important for experienced therapy companion dogs to **closely observe their behavior in the context of therapy** and to recognize early on when new behaviors appear in the dog's behavioral repertoire due to participant contact. Usually, these are—from the therapist's point of view—rather unwanted behaviors. If these are recognized early, they can usually be reduced again with appropriate training. In the following, I describe this aspect as well as the other aspects of preparation in more detail.

6.3.2.1 Dog Learns to Focus on the Participant

Perhaps the most fundamental behavior that a therapy companion dog should show is that it focuses on the participant during therapy. Conversely, this means that the dog should not focus on its reference person, the therapist, during therapy. The attention of the therapy companion dog should mainly be on the participant.

First, I would like to briefly explain why this is so important for therapy. After that, I will explain how this behavior is taught to the dog.

6.3.2.1.1 Important for All Forms of Animal-Assisted Therapy

The dog's ability to focus on the participant is important for any form of animal-assisted therapy and for any content exercise. Whether physical contact is made with the dog, the dog is observed, or active work is done with the dog—the point of animal-assisted therapy is that the participant and the dog are interacting with each other. For example, if the dog constantly only looks at the therapist and interacts with the participant only at the therapist's command, then neither relationship work nor therapy is possible. The dog must perceive the participant, react to him, interact with him. Only then is the basis for animal-assisted therapy established.

For the therapist, this means the following challenges: being able to *let go of the dog* and *hold back oneself*. The point of therapy is not to show how good one's own relationship with the dog is or how well the dog reacts to one. If someone has this aspiration, they should definitely abandon it. The therapist must be so sure of himself and the good relationship with his dog that he can easily let go of the dog and send it into interaction with other people. And if the dog also feels secure in the relationship with the therapist, then it will also easily and curiously approach other people.

▶   **Important!** The therapist must be so sure of himself and the good relationship with his dog that he can easily let go of the dog and send it into interaction with other people.

It should be clear at this point that this does not mean that the dog should necessarily be in unconditionally positive interaction with the participant. On the contrary, it should react authentically to the participant's behavior. This can also mean, for example, that it keeps a distance from the participant because he is crowding it. In order to be able to react authentically, however, the dog must first focus its attention on the participant.

6.3.2.1.2 Specific Training

The foundation for this is the *secure attachment between therapist and dog*. The dog must feel safe and comfortable with the therapist, and the therapist must feel safe and comfortable with the dog. There is a mutual bond of trust and respect. This foundation is so essential because the same processes occur as in the attachment between parents and child: If the child (the dog) is securely attached to its caregiver (the therapist), the child (the dog) can develop good self-confidence and a healthy curiosity. Self-confidence and curiosity, in turn, make the child (the dog) open to forming new relationships. In this context, one can also use the metaphor of a ship with a safe harbor: A ship that knows of a consistently safe harbor dares to venture into foreign waters.

Establishing a secure attachment with a dog takes some time. However, it is a misconception to think that this is automatically dependent on the age of the dog or the length of cohabitation. Dogs quickly learn which human provides them with security and the opportunity to trust and who does not. Thus, dogs that have lived with a human from puppyhood can be insecurely attached to them if they are given too little structure, security, or love. And just as quickly, a trusting and secure bond can be established with an adopted adult dog if it is given love, security, and structure. Nevertheless, it should be the case that the dog has already lived with one for between one and two years before there is a sufficiently secure relationship basis for joint work in animal-assisted therapy.

Once the secure attachment between therapist and dog is established, the dog can be actively taught to focus on the participant during therapy. This requires people who are willing to act as participants. With these, therapy settings are now simulated. Successively, the therapist withdraws from contact with the dog. Specifically, this means:

- not speaking to the dog on their own initiative
- not reacting to the dog when it comes and wants to be petted
- having the participant in focus themselves (because a securely attached dog is usually also interested in what interests its human!)

This should not happen abruptly to the dog, but slowly, so that the dog does not associate negative emotions with the therapy setting. One should also proceed at the dog's pace, i.e., observe how it reacts when it is *let go* and thus sent into interaction with others. Does it sadly lie down in its place or does it simply try its luck with the person who is mimicking the participant? The latter is the goal and if it occurs, the dog should be immediately reinforced by rewarding it with attention and affection from the person.

Most dogs quickly understand with this approach that they should focus not on the therapist, but on the participant in the therapy setting. Practicing in this case is therefore quite simple and entertaining.

However, it should be emphasized again at this point that the therapist's attitude is essential for success: As a therapist, I must be *sure* of myself and my relationship with the dog in order to enjoy the dog building relationships with others. Those who struggle internally with letting go of the dog, who feel jealousy or the desire to make their own relationship with the dog visible to others, should first deal with this. It can be helpful to ask oneself why it is difficult to let go of the dog. Am I insecure? Do I doubt my relationship with the dog? Do I feel the need to prove myself? Above all else, this personal insecurity should be resolved and a secure bond with the dog should be established. Because: Only a secure team consisting of a securely attached dog and a secure therapist can offer good animal-assisted therapy.

6.3.2.2 Dog Learns to Authentically Respond to the Participant's Behavior

This is by far the most important aspect of training—at the same time, it is also the aspect that cannot be trained with specific exercises. Because the dog is not actively taught a specific behavior here, but is *encouraged to be itself*. What does this mean in concrete terms?

A good therapy companion dog should react confidently and authentically to its counterpart. It should show whether it feels comfortable with someone or whether it prefers to keep a distance from this person. Because only in this way does the person receive honest feedback about their own impact and behavior. And only on this basis can therapeutic work be done on issues such as relationship building, social competence, and self-confidence in dealing with others. A participant who may repeatedly encounter rejection or dismissal in everyday life and cannot explain the reason for this, first needs feedback on their external impact before they can actively change anything. That's why the authentic behavior of the dogs is so important for therapy. They react bluntly and directly to the participant's behavior and reflect it through their reactions. My task then is to put their reactions into words and relate them to the participant's behavior.

Example: Authentic reactions of the dogs reflect the participant's own behavior

Participant 8 comes to the dog-assisted self-confidence training with a damaged self-esteem. She reports various humiliations and injuries in her professional and private environment. She feels rejected by various people and therefore devalues herself strongly.

In the interaction with Giulio, Participant 8 is initially friendly and attentive, but becomes demanding in the second session: Giulio comes to greet her, sits next to the participant and lets himself be petted, and then after a few minutes gets up to lie down on his resting place. Participant 8 tries to hold him back so that Giulio stays close to her. But Giulio is not deterred and goes to his resting place anyway. Participant 8 reports on request that she would like to call Giulio back or go over to him. I tell Participant 8 that she is encroaching on Giulio when she tries to force closeness to him. On this basis, we can discuss and practice the appropriate regulation of closeness and distance to Giulio. At the same time, I encourage the participant to view her interpersonal relationships from this perspective. Over time, it becomes clear that Participant 8 tries to force closeness in some relationships by encroaching on her counterpart or trying to exert emotional pressure on them. Some people then responded with contact termination or withdrawal, which Participant 8 initially could not directly relate to her own behavior.

Giulio's authentic reaction mirrored Participant 8 her own behavior. Giulio's honest and immediate reaction to the participant's behavior was thus the starting point for therapeutic work on the participant's general social competence. ◄

So, how do I promote the authentic reactions of my dogs?

My entire training with the dogs, the design of our shared leisure time, and my daily cohabitation with them aim to promote and preserve the *well-being* and thus the *self-confidence* of my dogs. Because: a dog that feels completely comfortable is self-confident. A dog that is self-confident behaves authentically.

In short words, this seems to be a fairly simple matter. But it is not. I always keep an eye on how the dogs are doing and what they need. What a situation does to them and how an interaction affects them. My entire life, thus not only my time at work, is always aimed at keeping my dogs in balance. To create balance, to offer them positive experiences and to bring relaxation into their everyday life. Maintaining the well-being and self-confidence of dogs that deal with psychiatric patients and mentally stressed participants on a daily basis, over years, is a very comprehensive and challenging task. I have to be flexible in dealing with changing circumstances and situations, always be ready to act and always have the dogs' well-being in mind.

▶   **Important!** For a therapy companion dog to behave authentically, it must feel **completely comfortable and self-confident as a dog**.
     The therapist's task is therefore the constant promotion and preservation of the dog's well-being and self-confidence!

Here are some specific ways to promote a dog's well-being and self-confidence:

• The dog should be kept physically fit and agile. Because *mens sana in corpore sano*—a healthy mind resides in a healthy body—applies not only to humans, but especially to dogs. For a dog to feel comfortable and secure in its own body, it needs healthy muscles, a good sense of balance, and good stamina. These can be trained, for example, through *extensive hikes, romping with other dogs*, and specific playful exercises during walks, such as *balancing* over tree trunks or *jumps* over ditches (see Fig. 6.8).
• The dog should feel comfortable in its family and with the other dogs it may live with. Here, it should be *sure of its role and position*, which is clarified by considering a clear hierarchy in dealing with the dogs (see Sect. 3.2.3). A matter of course, but worth mentioning again due to its importance, is the *consistently positive and loving treatment* of the dog (see Sect. 6.1).
• The dog should have a *structured daily routine* that gives it security, and at the same time, it should also experience something *new* again and again. Small adventures in nature, new experiences, and encounters are good ways to maintain the dog's *curiosity* and make it more confident by *successfully mastering small challenges*.
• The dog should be given the possibility to experience *regular small and large successes*. This can be as simple as the noodle that fell in the kitchen that the dog "secretly snatches" or the successfully completed search exercise during the walk. Of course, not constantly and for every little thing, but still, a *enthusiastic praise* is an important source of self-confidence for the dog. Because hearing, seeing, and feeling that his reference person reacts enthusiastically to him is a beautiful and above all strengthening experience for the dog.
• The dog should be actively encouraged to relax physically and mentally. Certain *massage techniques* can be helpful here, as can the conscious creation of a *calm and relaxed atmosphere*.

Fig. 6.8 Keeping dogs physically fit and agile—jumps and balancing in the forest are a good way to do this

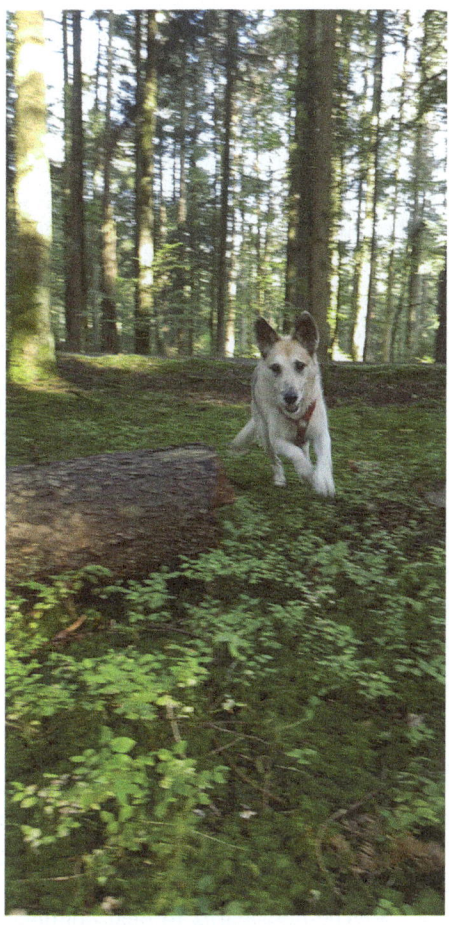

6.3.2.3 Dog Learns to Deal Confidently with Various People

Essential to the training of the dog in preparation for its deployment as a therapy companion dog is the gathering of experiences with different people. Here, the dog should not only meet many people, but above all as many different groups of people as possible. So not just many different healthy adults, but also teenagers, children, older people, women and men, and so on. It is important that the interaction with people is positively associated for the dog, brings him joy, and at the same time does not overwhelm him.

When I began working with Giulio years ago, I had the best conditions for it. Through my work as a psychologist at a psychosomatic clinic, I was able to introduce Giulio to many different people at the beginning of his deployment. Initially, he was simply present during the individual conversations I had with patients as a therapist. When I noticed how positively the patients reacted to his presence, I took him into group therapies and gradually developed my animal-assisted therapy concept based on the experiences made there (see Sect. 1.3.1).

During this time, Giulio got to know a wide variety of people: young and old, heavily burdened and resilient, women and men. People with personality disorders, anxiety disorders, pain disorders, autonomic dysfunctions, and depressive illnesses. People with physical limitations and disabilities. People in suicidal crises. People during a radical upheaval in their lives. Open and friendly people and closed, bitter people. People who love dogs, and people with a dog phobia.

There were very, very many different people that Giulio got to know. It was important for his initial development that he could actively regulate contact with them himself. He was present in the room while I conducted the therapeutic conversations with the patients and could decide at any time whether he wanted to approach the patient or not. Since Giulio is very sociable, he usually came to the patients, sat next to them, and let himself be petted. However, I noticed differences in his reactions to the patients' conditions.

And this is the second reason why contact with many different people is so important in preparing the dog: On the one hand, as mentioned, the dog learns to deal confidently with different people and gets used to the groups of people he will have to deal with in his work as a therapy support dog. On the other hand, the therapist makes important observations regarding the dog's authentic reactions. These are, as previously described (see Sect. 5.1.4), essential for therapeutic work. Only if I as a therapist know exactly how my dog reacts to emotions and behaviors, can I read his reactions to a participant and draw conclusions from these reactions about the participant's condition and effect. These observations and analyses, in turn, are the essential basis of my dog-supported self-confidence training.

▶   **Important!** The dog's acclimatization to dealing with different people is a significant part of preparing a therapy support dog for two important reasons:

1. The dog learns to deal confidently with the later participants in animal-assisted therapy
2. The therapist learns how the dog reacts to different people and especially to different emotions and behaviors

The background to this is: Only if the therapist knows exactly how his dog reacts to emotions and behaviors, can he read the dog's reactions in the context of animal-assisted therapy and draw conclusions from the reactions about the participant's condition and effect.

During this initial phase of Giulio and I working together with the patients of the psychosomatic clinic, I made the following observations:

• If a patient was sad, Giulio sought proximity to him
• If a patient was very tense, Giulio kept his distance
• If a patient was nervous or upset, Giulio became restless

- If a patient was relaxed, Giulio slept deeply and soundly

And the patient's behavior also determined the contact with Giulio:

- If a patient wanted to force closeness to Giulio, Giulio resisted
- If a patient was benevolent and open, he quickly had the most intimate contact with Giulio (see Fig. 6.9)

For a more detailed description of Giulio's reactions to the patients' conditions, I refer to the relevant article on the subject (Blesch, 2015).

During this initial phase of getting to know various people intensively, I accepted and reinforced Giulio's individual reactions. In this way, I trained not only the habituation to dealing with various people but also the authenticity of his behavior. And, as I said, I learned more and more about Giulio's reactions to human moods and behaviors.

It should be noted at this point how closely intertwined the individual aspects of preparation and training are. Everything is interconnected and builds on each other. And especially when getting to know various people, it is important to use these situations to convey to the dog that he is allowed to behave authentically according to his feelings.

▶   **Important!** In preparing dogs for their use in therapy, all learning experiences and training steps are closely interconnected. Various aspects (accli-

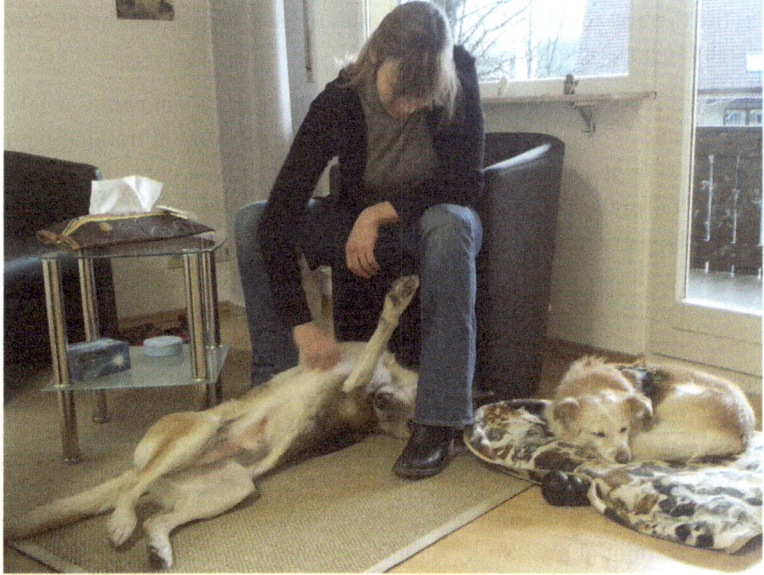

Fig. 6.9 When Giulio feels comfortable with someone, this trusting, proximity-seeking position is typical for him

mating the dog to different people; promoting the dog's authenticity; conveying basic rules; getting to know the dog better; and so on) merge into each other and often develop in parallel and build upon each other.

6.3.2.4 Lifelong Learning also for Fully Trained Therapy Dogs

As initially described on this topic (see Sect. 6.3.2) and as also made clear elsewhere (sections on *taking breaks*, *creating balance* and *practicing self-criticism* in Sect. 3.4), the animal-assisted work with a therapy dog is not self-sustaining even after its training. Rather, it is necessary to continuously work on maintaining his well-being and thus his operational readiness in everyday life. In addition, it should be vigilantly observed how the contact with the participants changes the dog in his reactions.

At the beginning, I described the influence of the participants on the dog's reactions with the image of the constant drip that hollows out the stone over time. And that's exactly how it is. Years of patient or participant contact also influences a routine and balanced therapy companion dog. And so it can happen that the dog exhibits unwanted behaviors during the course of his deployment in therapy, as he is reinforced by the participants in some way. Therefore, even after the dog's preparation for his deployment as a therapy companion dog is completed, it is important to vigilantly observe his behavior in the context of therapy and to recognize early on when new behaviors appear in the dog's behavioral repertoire due to participant contact or the therapy setting.

As the example shows, it doesn't always have to be something dramatic, it can also be something quite amusing that the dog suddenly exhibits in new behaviors.

> **Example: The therapy companion dog continues to learn throughout his life—even after his training is completed!**
>
> As described, a session with me goes as follows: the participant comes and we discuss his current condition and the specific content of the subsequent training with the dog. This is followed by the training. At the end of the session, a debriefing of the training takes place. During the debriefing, the dogs usually lie on one of their resting places or sit next to the participant and let themselves be petted.
>
> There was a phase when Giulio would jump up during the debriefing and run to the door as soon as he heard me say the word "So …". I still have to laugh about it today when I think about it. He had learned that I initiated the end of the therapy session with a "So …". I wasn't even aware of this fact myself at first. I only realized it when Giulio started to get up and go to the door whenever I said "So …". Now, this was primarily an amusing behavior that Giulio had acquired, because it made me smile about myself and my predictability for Giulio. However, I didn't want this behavior to become permanently ingrained in Giulio, because his sudden getting up and going to the door at my "So …" could seem like ushering out the participant. So I weaned Giulio off this behavior by consciously paying attention to my own behavior. I consciously avoided saying "So…" at the end of the session and instead sprinkled

the word in at other times (it was important here that I also used the same drawn-out emphasis of the word that I—as I had learned from Giulio—apparently always used at the end of the session), to convey to him that this word had no meaning for him. Giulio quickly unlearned the habit of ushering out the participants. Every now and then he still looks at me very closely when the word "So …" slips out at the end of a session, and I usually have to laugh to myself. It has become somewaht our secret "running gag". ◄

These newly acquired, unwanted behaviors of the dog can therefore be minor things or something amusing, or they can also be something that actually disrupts or negatively influences the therapy process. The dog must therefore always be observed attentively, even after years. If you observe the dog and do not take his good behavior for granted, you will recognize early on when an unwanted behavior develops. And the earlier such behaviors are recognized, the faster and easier they can be eliminated with appropriate training.

References

Blesch, K. (2015). Tiergestützte Gruppenpsychotherapie. *Gruppenpsychotherapie—Gruppendynamik, 51,* 86–97.
Fiss-Quelle, S. (2016). *Faktor Mensch—Kundenkommunikation und Konfliktlösung für Hundeprofis.* Kynos.
Ullrich, A. (2016). *Impulskontrolle—Wie Hunde sich beherrschen lernen.* MenschHund.
Wischall-Wagner, A. (2019). *Entspannter Mensch—Entspannter Hund … so glückt das Zusammenleben wie von selbst.* Gräfe & Unzer.

Afterword

7

Abstract

This final, brief chapter represents a personal obituary in one's own cause.

During the work on this book, Cleo passed away. She fell seriously ill shortly after her retirement and never fully recovered despite lengthy and intensive treatments and care. For several months, she continued to live her life with pleasure despite her illness and increasing frailty, but gradually became weaker until she finally had to be put to sleep with a heavy heart.

Unfortunately, the final phase of life and the death of the dog are also part of living and working with dogs. Making this difficult journey as easy as possible for the dog, despite one's own grief, is the last opportunity to be there for the beloved dog at the end of their shared life. And I am grateful that this was possible, and Cleo was able to leave peacefully. Particularly touching was the behavior of Giulio and Toni. Both were especially loving with Cleo in the last weeks and did not leave her side on her last day (see Fig. 7.1).

And what remains are the memories, the gratitude for the shared years, and the traces of change and development that Cleo initiated and accompanied in me and in other people. The same applies to my other deceased dogs, who were part of my life and will continue to be part of my life in the form of thoughts and memories. No dog leaves a person as they were—if the person engages in the relationship with the dog.

And so I quote again, this time freely, the natural philosopher John Muir: *Every insight into the life of an animal enriches our own life and makes it wider and better in every respect.*

K. Blesch, *Animal-Assisted Therapy with Dogs*, https://doi.org/10.1007/978-3-662-67965-4_7

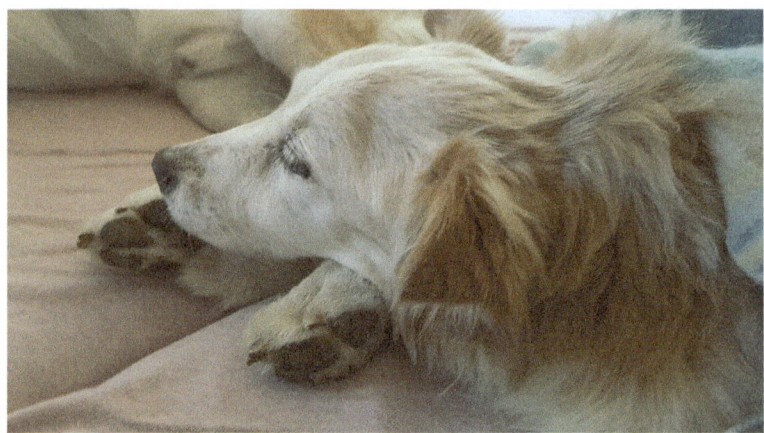

Fig. 7.1 Together until the end—Cleo spent her last hours lying on Giulio's paws

Further Reading

Auslitz-Blesch, K. (2015). *Pepe, the artist of life—A small dog gets his life back.* R.G. Fischer.

Blesch, R. W., & Mödinger, W. (2014). Dialogic Leadership—A Contribution to the Legitimization of Future-Oriented Leadership. *International Journal for Philosophy and Psychosomatics, 2,* 1–13.

Cavalieri, P. (2002). *The question of animals—For an expanded theory of human rights.* Harald Fischer.

ESAAT. ESAAT Principles. As pdf-download at www.esaat.org. Accessed: 19. Dec. 2019.

Falconer-Taylor, R., Neville, P., & Strong, V. (2013). *Assessing emotions, understanding dogs.* Cadmos.

Liechti, M. (Ed.). (2002). *The dignity of animals.* Harald Fischer.

Meijer, E. (2018). *The languages of animals.* Matthes & Seitz.

Humans for Animal Rights. (2018). www.tierrechte.de/2018/07/11/interview-der-mensch-missachtet-die-grundbeduerfnisse-der-pferde/. Accessed: 26. July 2019.

Müller, C. A., Schmitt, K., Barber, A. L., & Huber, L. (2015). Dogs can discriminate emotional expressions of human faces. *Current Biology, 25,* 601–605.

Olbrich, E., Beetz, A., & Julius, H. (2008). Elements of a theory of human-animal relationship. In Grosse-Siestrup et al. (Eds.), *Congress Human and Animal—Animals in Prevention and Therapy 2008* (p. 160). http://www.mensch-tier-kongress.de. Accessed: 26. July 2019.

Topál, J., Gásci, M., Miklósi, A., Virányi, Z., Kubinyi, E., & Csányi, V. (2005). Attachment to humans: A comparative study on hand-reared wolves and differently socialized dog puppies. *Animal Behavior, 70*(6), 1367–1375.

Wanser, S. H., & Udell, M. A. R. (2019). Does attachment security to a human handler influence the behavior of dogs who engage in animal assisted activities? *Applied animal behavior science, 210,* 88–94.

Wolf, J. C. (2005). *Animal ethics—New perspectives for humans and animals.* Harald Fischer.

Central Association of Zoological Specialist Businesses in Germany e. V. (2018). www.zzf.de. Accessed: 12. July 2019.

The manufacturer's authorised representative in the EU is Springer
Nature Customer Service Centre GmbH, Europaplatz 3, 69115 Heidelberg,
Germany. If you have any concerns regarding our products, please
contact ProductSafety@springernature.com

Printed and bound by CPI Group (UK) Ltd, Croydon, CR0 4YY
24/04/2026
02096366-0007